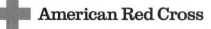
American Red Cross

C O M M U N I T Y
FIRST AID &
SAFETY

Important certification information

American Red Cross certificates may be issued upon successful
completion of a training program that uses this textbook as an
integral part of the course. By itself, the text material does not constitute comprehensive Red Cross training. In order to issue ARC certificates, your instructor must be authorized by the American Red Cross
and must follow prescribed policies and procedures. Make certain that
you have attended a course authorized by the Red Cross. Ask your
instructor about receiving American Red Cross certification, or contact
your local chapter for more information.

✚ **American Red Cross**

C O M M U N I T Y
FIRST AID &
SAFETY

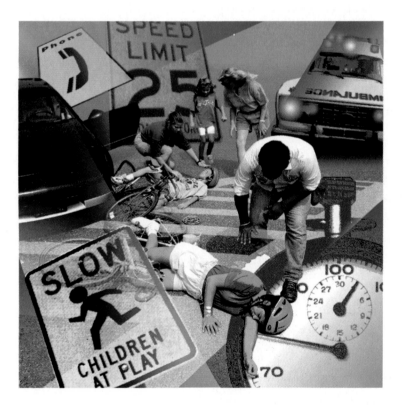

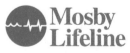 Mosby
Lifeline

St. Louis Baltimore Boston Chicago London Philadelphia Sydney Toronto

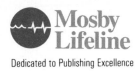
Dedicated to Publishing Excellence

This participant's textbook is an integral part of
American Red Cross training. By itself, it does not constitute complete
and comprehensive training.

The emergency care procedures outlined in this book reflect the
standard of knowledge and accepted emergency practices in the
United States at the time this book was published. It is the reader's
responsibility to stay informed of changes in the emergency
care procedures.

Printed in the United States of America.

Mosby Lifeline
Mosby–Year Book, Inc.
11830 Westline Industrial Drive
St. Louis, MO 63146

Library of Congress Cataloging in Publication Data

Community first aid and safety / American Red Cross.
    p.   cm.
  Includes index.
  ISBN 0-8016-7064-0
  1. First aid in illness and injury.   I. American Red Cross.
RC86.7.C644 1993   92-585
616.02'52—dc20   CIP

95 96 97 CL/CD/BA 9

ACKNOWLEDGEMENTS

This course and participant's manual were developed and produced through a joint effort of the American Red Cross and the Mosby–Year Book Publishing Company. Many individuals shared in the overall process in supportive, technical, and creative ways. This manual could not have been developed without the dedication of both paid and volunteer staff. Their commitment to excellence made this manual possible.

The Health and Safety Program Development staff at American Red Cross national headquarters responsible for the instructional design and writing of this course and manual included: Lawrence D. Newell, EdD, NREMT-P, Project Manager; Martha F. Beshers; Thomas J.S. Edwards, PhD; M. Elizabeth Buoy-Morrissey, MPH; Robert T. Ogle; and S. Elizabeth White, MAEd, ATC, Associates; Sandra D. Buesking, Lori M. Compton, Marian F.H. Kirk, and O. Paul Stearns, Analysts. Administrative support was provided by Denise Beale and Ella Holloway.

The following American Red Cross national headquarters Health and Safety volunteer and paid staff provided guidance and review: Robert F. Burnside, Director; Frank Carroll, Manager, Program Development; Richard M. Walter, Manager, Operations; and Stephen Silverman, EdD, National Volunteer Consultant for Program Development.

The Mosby Lifeline publishing team based in Hanover, Maryland, included: David Culverwell, Vice President and Publisher; Claire Merrick, Senior Editor; Richard Weimer, Executive Editor; and Dana Battaglia, Assistant Editor.

The Mosby–Year Book Editorial and Production Team based in St. Louis, Missouri, included: Virgil Mette, Executive Vice President; Carol Sullivan Wiseman, Project Manager; Diana Lyn Laulainen, Production Editor; Kay Kramer, Director of Art and Design; Jerry A. Wood, Director of Manufacturing; Patricia Stinecipher, Special Product Manager; and Kathy Grone, Manufacturing Supervisor.

Special thanks go to Rick Brady, Photographer and Kathy Barkey, Designer.

Guidance and review were also provided by the members of the American Red Cross CPR/First Aid Advisory Group including:

Ray Cranston
Chairperson
Commanding Officer, Traffic Safety Unit
Farmington Hills Police Department
Farmington Hills, Michigan

Larry Bair
Director, Health and Safety and Tissue Services
Central Iowa Chapter
Des Moines, Iowa

John E. Hendrickson
Director, Safety and Health
Mid-America Chapter
Chicago, Illinois

Andra Jones
Director, Health and Safety
Central Mississippi Chapter
Jackson, Mississippi

Sherri Olson-Roberts
Director, Health and Safety
Washtenaw County Chapter
Ann Arbor, Michigan

James A. Otte
Chairman, Health and Safety Committee
Glynn County Chapter
Brunswick, Georgia

Teresita B. Ramirez
Centex County Chapter
Lecturer, Department of Curriculum and Instruction
The University of Texas at Austin
Austin, Texas

W. Douglas Round
Captain, Greeley Fire Department
Colorado Territory
Greeley, Colorado

Natalie Lynne Smith, MS
Greater Hartford Chapter
Farmington, Connecticut

Linda S. Wenger
Director, Health and Safety
Lancaster County Chapter
Lancaster, Pennsylvania

David J. Wurzer, PhD
Greater Long Beach Chapter
Long Beach, California

External review was provided by the following organizations and individuals:

Gloria M. Blatti, RN, FNP, EdD
Adelphi University
Long Island, New York

Nisha C. Chandra, MD
Division of Cardiology
Francis Scott Key Medical Center
Baltimore, Maryland

Loring S. Flint, MD
Vice President
Baystate Medical Center
Springfield, Massachusetts

Robert C. Luten, MD
Director, Pediatric EMS
University of Florida
Health Science Center—Jacksonville
Jacksonville, Florida

John A. Paraskos, MD
Associate Director of C.V. Medicine
University of Massachusetts, Medical School
Worcester, Massachusetts

James S. Seidel, MD, PhD
Associate Professor of UCLA
Chief, Ambulatory Pediatrics
Torrance, California

Jay Shaw
Associate Professor
Eastern Montana College
American Red Cross Midland Empire Chapter
Board of Directors, Supervisory Committee
Billings, Montana

Edward Stapleton, EMT-P
Department of Emergency Medicine
Health Sciences Center
State University of New York at Stony Brook
Stony Brook, New York

ABOUT THIS COURSE

People need to know what to do in an emergency before medical help arrives. Since you may be faced with an emergency in your lifetime, it's important that you know how to recognize an emergency and how to respond. The intent of this course is to help people feel more confident of their ability to act appropriately in the event of an emergency.

After you complete this course, we believe you will be able to—
• Identify ways to prevent injury and/or illness.
• Recognize when an emergency has occurred.
• Follow three emergency action steps in any emergency.
• Provide basic care for injury and/or sudden illness until the victim can receive professional medical help.

To help you achieve this goal, you will read information in this manual, view a series of video segments, and participate in a number of learning activities designed to increase your knowledge and skills.

In addition, this course emphasizes the value of a safe and healthy life-style. It attempts to alert you to behavior and situations that contribute to your risk of injury and/or illness and to motivate you to take precautions and make any necessary life-style changes.

This manual contains all the material you learn in class in a form you can keep and refer to whenever you wish. Highlighted information and material condensed in lists make it easy for you to identify the critical points and to refresh your memory quickly. Photos, drawings, graphs, and tables also present information in an easy-to-find form. Skill sheets give step-by-step directions for performing the skills taught in the course. Questionnaires provide a way for you to evaluate certain risks in your life-style. Articles of varying lengths cover all the topics taught. Features contain information that enhances the information in the articles.

You may be taking this course not only because you feel a need to learn what to do if faced with an emergency but because of a job requirement specifying that you complete training and achieve a specific level of competency on both skill and written evaluations. In this case the American Red Cross provides a course completion certificate. You will be eligible to receive a certificate if you—
• Perform specific skills competently and demonstrate the ability to make appropriate decisions for care.
• Pass a final written exam with a score of 80 percent or higher.

If you do not have a requirement to achieve a specific level of competency on both skill and written evaluations, you will not need a course completion certificate. You will also not need to take the final examination for a passing score.

HEALTH PRECAUTIONS AND GUIDELINES DURING TRAINING

The American Red Cross has trained millions of people in first aid and CPR (cardiopulmonary resuscitation), using manikins as training aids. According to the Centers for Disease Control (CDC), there has never been a documented case of any disease caused by bacteria, a fungus, or a virus transmitted through the use of training aids, such as manikins used for CPR.

The American Red Cross follows widely accepted guidelines for cleaning and decontaminating training manikins. **If these guidelines are adhered to, the risk of any kind of disease transmission during training is extremely low.**

To help minimize the risk of disease transmission, you should follow some basic health precautions and guidelines while participating in training. You should take precautions if you have a condition that would increase your risk or other participants' risk of exposure to infections. Request a separate training manikin if you—

• Have an acute condition, such as a cold, a sore throat, or cuts or sores on your hands or around your mouth.

• Know you are seropositive (have had a positive blood test) for hepatitis B surface antigen (HBsAg), indicating that you are currently infected with the hepatitis B virus.*

• Know you have a chronic infection indicated by long-term seropositivity (long-term positive blood tests) for hepatitis B surface antigen (HBsAg)* or a positive blood test for anti–HIV (that is, a positive test for antibodies to HIV, the virus that causes many severe infections including AIDS).

• Have a type of condition that makes you unusually likely to get an infection.

*A person with hepatitis B infection will test positive for the hepatitis B surface antigen (HBsAg). Most persons infected with hepatitis B will get better within a period of time. However, some hepatitis B infections will become chronic and linger for much longer. These persons will continue to test positive for HBsAg. Their decision to participate in CPR training should be guided by their physician.
After a person has had an acute hepatitis B infection, he or she will no longer test positive for the surface antigen but will test positive for the hepatitis B antibody (anti-HBs). Persons who have been vaccinated for hepatitis B will also test positive for the hepatitis B antibody. A positive test for the hepatitis B antibody (anti-HBs) should not be confused with a positive test for the hepatitis B surface antigen (HBsAg).

If you decide you should have your own manikin, ask your instructor if he or she can provide one for you to use. You will not be asked to explain why in your request. The manikin will not be used by anyone else until it has been cleaned according to the recommended end-of-class decontamination procedures. The number of manikins available for class use is limited. Therefore the more advance notice you give, the more likely it is that you can be provided a separate manikin.

In addition to taking the precautions regarding manikins, you can further protect yourself and other participants from infection by following these guidelines:

• Wash your hands thoroughly before participating in class activities.

• Do not eat, drink, use tobacco products, or chew gum during classes when manikins are used.

• Clean the manikin properly before use. For some manikins, this means vigorously wiping the manikin's face and the inside of its mouth with a clean gauze pad soaked with either a solution of liquid chlorine bleach and water (sodium hypochlorite and water) or rubbing alcohol. For other manikins, it means changing the rubber face. Your instructor will provide you with instructions for cleaning the type of manikin used in your class.

• Follow the guidelines provided by your instructor when practicing skills such as clearing a blocked airway with your finger.

Training in first aid and CPR requires physical activity. If you have a medical condition or disability that will prevent you from taking part in the practice sessions, please let your instructor know.

CONTENTS

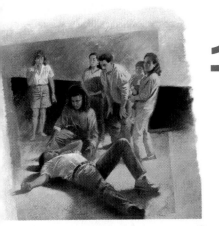

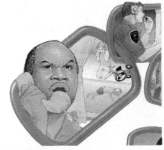

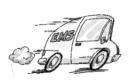

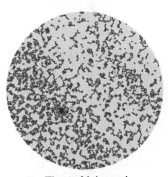

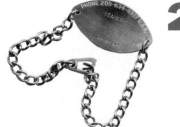

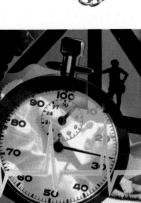

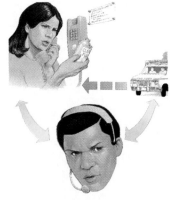

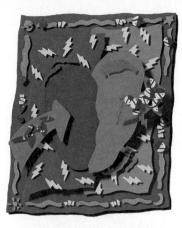

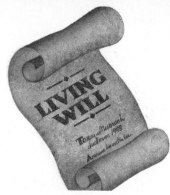

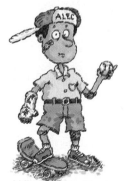

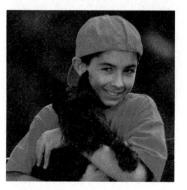

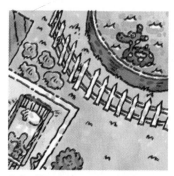

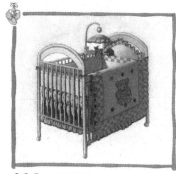

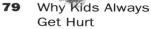

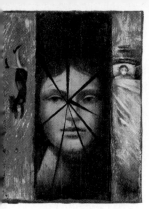

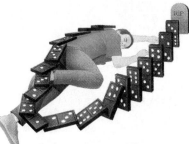

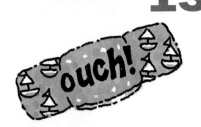

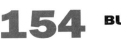

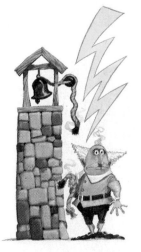

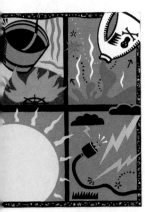

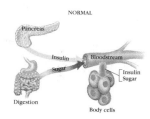

NORMAL

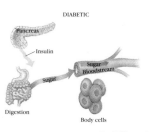

DIABETIC

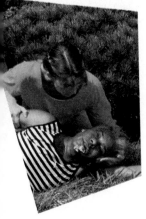

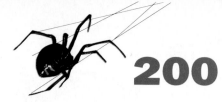

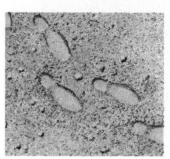

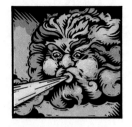

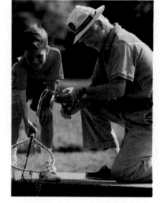

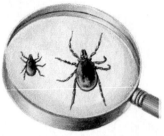

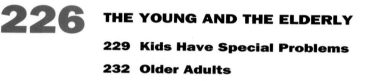

SKILL SHEETS

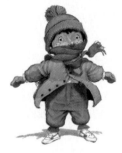

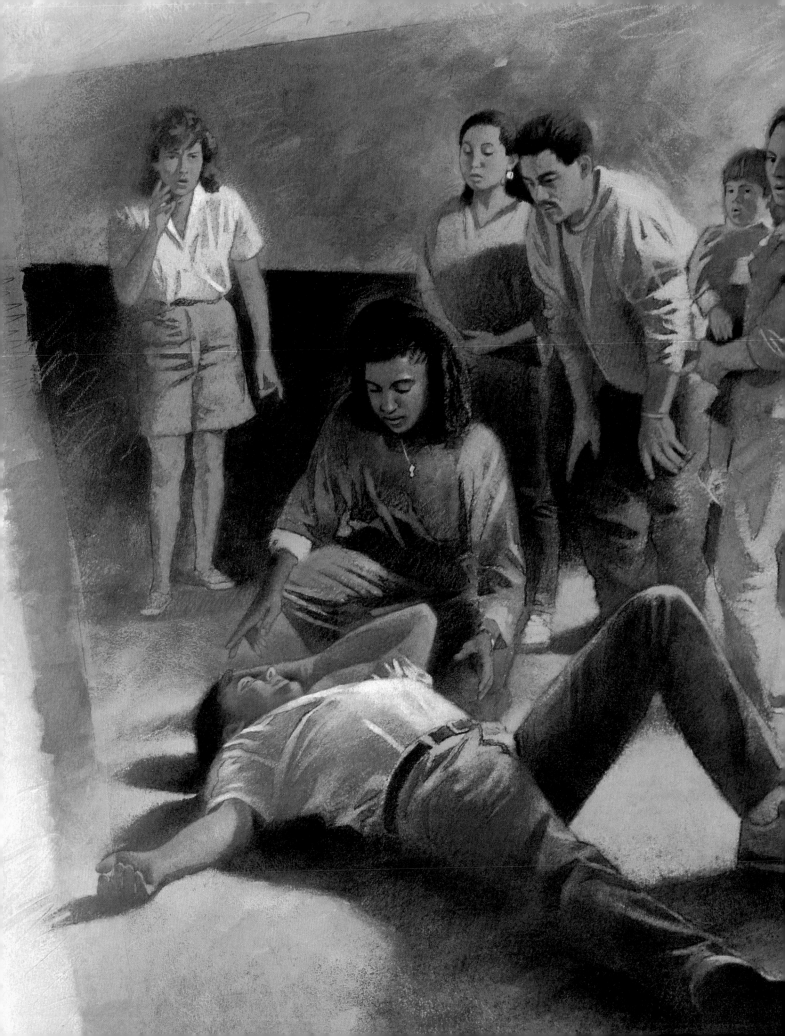

Why did you say you'd get to the party by seven o'clock? It's a good thing you stopped at the convenience store now and not later. Only a couple of things to buy. Why are all those people standing around over there? Oh no! It's the person who works here. . . . You leave the car and see the young man lying on his back, looking dazed, and holding his head. Even though a crowd has gathered, no one is helping him. They are just looking at each other. He needs help from some-one. That someone could be you!

If not YOU... Who?

GET INVOLVED

If placed in the above situation, would you step forward to help? "I hope I never have to," is what you are probably saying to yourself. However, given the number of injuries and sudden illnesses that occur in the United States each year, you might well have to deal with an emergency situation someday.

Consider the following:

- About 2 million people are hospitalized each year because of injuries, and injuries result in nearly 142,500 deaths each year.

- Infectious diseases used to cause the greatest concern about the health of children, but now, unintentional injuries cause most childhood deaths. Injuries also cause millions of heart-stopping moments each year. In fact, injuries are the leading cause of death and disability in children and young adults.
- More than 70 million people in the United States have cardiovascular disease. Cardiovascular disease causes about 1 million deaths in the United States each year. That's nearly half of the deaths that occur each year!
- Over 500,000 Americans have strokes each year, and 150,000 Americans die each year from stroke.

Each time a person is injured or experiences a sudden illness, such as a heart attack or a stroke, someone has to do something to help. You may find yourself in the position of having to provide help someday.

Everyone should know what to do in an emergency. You should know who to call and what care to provide. Providing care involves giving first aid until professional medical help arrives. Everyone should know first aid, but even if you haven't had any first aid training, you can still help in an emergency.

Calling your local emergency phone number is the most important thing you can do. The sooner medical help arrives, the better a person's chances of surviving a life-threatening emergency. You play a

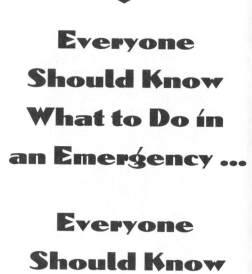

Everyone Should Know What to Do in an Emergency ...

Everyone Should Know First Aid.

major role in making the emergency medical services (EMS) system work effectively. The EMS system is a network of police, fire, and medical personnel, as well as other community resources.

Your role in the EMS system includes four basic steps:
1. *Recognize* that an emergency exists.
2. *Decide* to act.
3. *Call* the local emergency telephone number for help.
4. *Provide* care until help arrives.

Of course, steps 3 and 4 won't happen if you don't take steps 1 and 2. By recognizing an emergency and taking action to help,

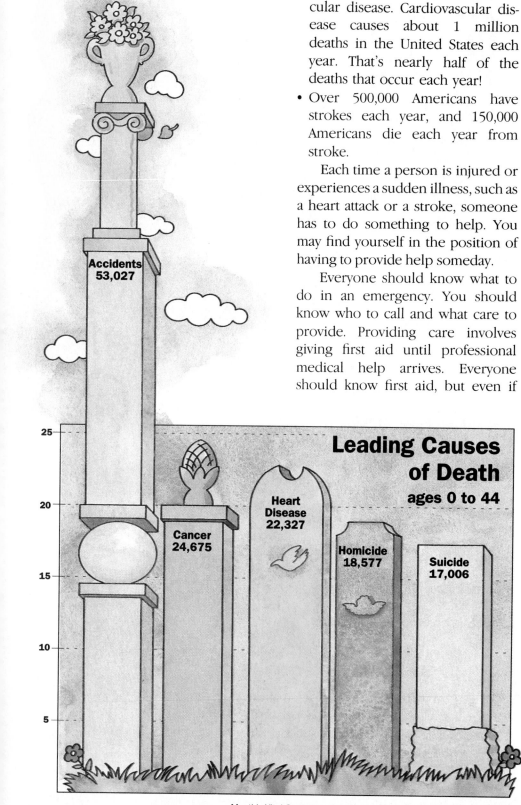

Leading Causes of Death

ages 0 to 44

Accidents
53,027

Cancer
24,675

Heart Disease
22,327

Homicide
18,577

Suicide
17,006

25 —
20 —
15 —
10 —
5 —

Monthly Vital Statistics. Vol. 40, No. 8, Supplement 2. Jan. 7, 1992.

1. Citizen Response

2. Calling the Emergency Number

3. First Responder Care

4. EMT Care

5. Hospital Care

6. Rehabilitation

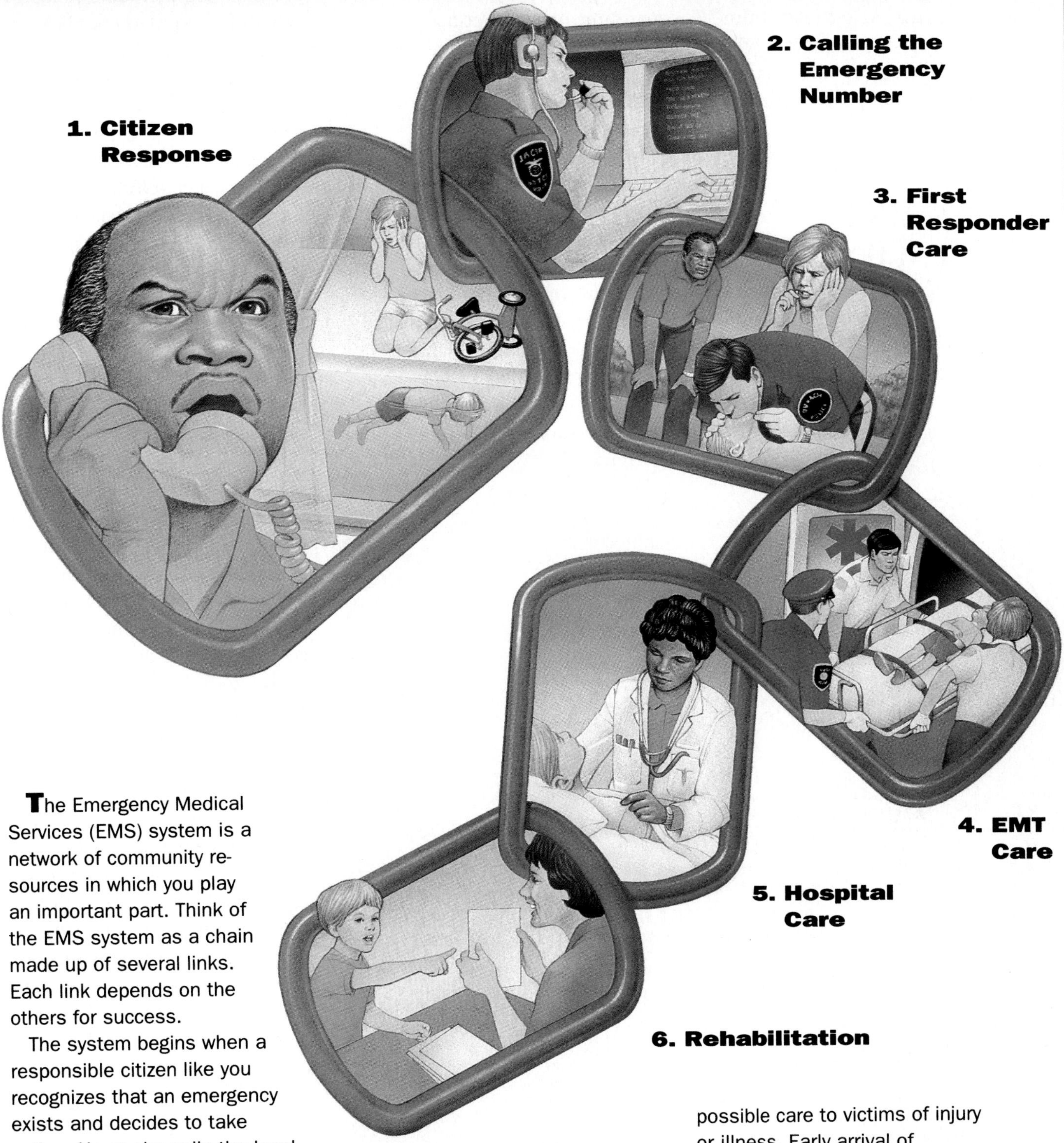

The Emergency Medical Services (EMS) system is a network of community resources in which you play an important part. Think of the EMS system as a chain made up of several links. Each link depends on the others for success.

The system begins when a responsible citizen like you recognizes that an emergency exists and decides to take action. He or she calls the local emergency number for help. The EMS dispatcher answers the call and uses the information you give to determine what help is needed. A team of emergency personnel gives care at the scene and transports the victim to the hospital where emergency department staff and a variety of other professionals take over.

Ideally, a victim will move through each link in the chain. All the links should work together to provide the best possible care to victims of injury or illness. Early arrival of emergency personnel increases the victim's chances of surviving a life-threatening emergency. Whether or not you know first aid, calling your emergency number is the most important action you can take.

you give injured or ill persons the best chance for survival. Know your local emergency telephone number. The rapid arrival of professional help increases the victim's chances of surviving a life-threatening emergency.

RECOGNIZING EMERGENCIES

Emergencies can happen to anyone and they can happen anywhere, but before you can give help you must be able to recognize an emergency. You may realize that an emergency has occurred only if something unusual attracts your attention. For example, you may become aware of unusual noises, sights, odors, and appearances or behaviors.

Noises that may signal an emergency include screaming or calls for help; breaking glass, crashing metal, or screeching tires; a change in the sound made by machinery or equipment; or sudden, loud noises, like those made by collapsing buildings or falling ladders or when a person falls.

Signals of an emergency that you may see include a person lying motionless, spilled chemicals, fallen boxes, a power failure or downed electrical wires, or smoke or fire.

Many odors are part of our everyday lives, for example, gasoline fumes at a gas station, the smell of chlorine at a swimming pool, and the smell of chemicals at a refinery. However, when these are stronger than usual, there may be an emergency. Also, an unusual odor may mean something is wrong. Put your own safety first. Leave the area if there is an unusual or very strong odor, since some fumes are poisonous.

It may be difficult to tell if someone is behaving strangely or if something is wrong, especially if you don't know the person. Some actions leave little doubt that something might be wrong. For example, if you see someone suddenly collapse or slip and fall, you have a fairly good idea that the person might need some help.

Other signals of a possible emergency might not be as easy to recognize. They include signals of breathing difficulty, confused behavior, unusual skin color, signs of pain or discomfort, such as clutching the chest or throat or being doubled over, or facial expressions indicating something is wrong.

Sometimes it is obvious that something is wrong; at other times it is more difficult to be sure. For example, a person having a heart attack may clutch his or her chest, begin to perspire, and have difficulty breathing. Another heart attack victim may only feel mild chest pain and not give any obvious signals of distress. The important thing is to recognize that an emergency might have occurred.

RECOGNIZING EMERGENCIES

Your senses—hearing, sight, and smell—may help you recognize an emergency. Emergencies are often signaled by something unusual that catches your attention.

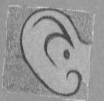

UNUSUAL NOISES
Screams, yells, moans, or calls for help
Breaking glass, crashing metal, or screeching tires
Changes in machinery or equipment noises
Sudden, loud voices

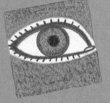

UNUSUAL SIGHTS
A stalled vehicle
An overturned pot
A spilled medicine container
Broken glass
Downed electrical wires
Smoke or fire

UNUSUAL ODORS
Odors that are stronger than usual
Unrecognizable odors

UNUSUAL APPEARANCES OR BEHAVIORS
Difficulty breathing
Clutching the chest or throat
Slurred, confused, or hesitant speech
Unexplainable confusion or drowsiness
Sweating for no apparent reason
Unusual skin color

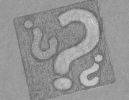

DECIDING TO ACT

Once you recognize an emergency has occurred, you must decide whether to help and how you can best help. There are many ways you can help in an emergency. *In order to help, you must act.*

▼

There are Many Ways to Help in an Emergency. In Order to Help, You Must Act.

Whether or not you have had first aid training, being faced with an emergency will probably cause you to have mixed feelings. Besides wanting to help, you may have other feelings that make you hesitate or back away from the situation. These feelings are personal and very real. The decision to act is yours and yours alone.

Sometimes, even though people recognize that what has happened is an emergency, they fail to act. There are many reasons why people don't act in an emergency. The most common factors that influence a person's response include—
• The presence of other people.
• Uncertainty about the victim.
• The type of injury or illness.

What Everyone Should Know About Good Samaritan Laws

Are there laws to protect you when you help in an emergency situation?

Yes, most states have enacted Good Samaritan laws. These laws give legal protection to people who provide emergency care to ill or injured persons.

When citizens respond to an emergency and act as a *reasonable* and *prudent* person would under the same conditions, Good Samaritan immunity generally prevails. This legal immunity protects you, as a rescuer, from being sued and found financially responsible for the victim's injury. For example, a reasonable and prudent person would—

■ Move a victim only if the victim's life was endangered.
■ Ask a conscious victim for permission before giving care.
■ Check the victim for life-threatening emergencies before providing further care.
■ Summon professional help to the scene by calling the local emergency number or the operator.
■ Continue to provide care until more highly trained personnel arrive.

Good Samaritan laws were developed to encourage people to help others in emergency situations. They require that the "Good Samaritan" use common sense and a reasonable level of skill, not to exceed the scope of the individual's training in emergency situations. They assume each person would do his or her best to save a life or prevent further injury.

People are rarely sued for helping in an emergency. However, the existence of Good Samaritan laws does not mean that someone cannot sue. In rare cases, courts have ruled that these laws do not apply in cases when an individual rescuer's response was grossly or willfully negligent or reckless or when the rescuer abandoned the victim after initiating care.

If you are interested in finding out about your state's Good Samaritan laws, contact a legal professional or check with your local library.

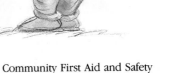

- Fear of catching a disease.
- Fear of doing something wrong.

If there are several people standing around, it might not be easy to tell if anyone is providing first aid. Always ask if you can help. Just because there is a crowd doesn't mean someone is caring for the victim. In fact, you may be the only one there who knows first aid.

Although you may feel embarrassed about coming forward in front of other people, this should not stop you from offering help. Someone has to take action in an emergency, and it may have to be you, even though you don't want to become the center of attention. If others are already giving care, ask if you can help.

If there are people around, but they do not appear to be helping, tell them how to help. You can ask them to call the emergency number, meet the ambulance and direct it to your location, keep the area free of onlookers and traffic, or help give care. You might send them for blankets or other supplies.

Most emergencies happen in or near the home, so you are more likely to give care to a family member or a friend than to someone you do not know. However, this isn't always the case. There may be a time when you do not know the victim and feel uneasy about helping a stranger. Sometimes you might not be sure about taking ac-

FIRST AID

Bacteria and viruses are common forms of germs.

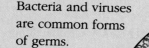

Streptococcus agalactia bacteria

You are driving home from work. Suddenly, you hear a crash. A person on a bike has been hit by a car and is bleeding. You want to help but are afraid. You ask yourself, "Will I catch a disease if I give first aid? How do diseases pass from one person to another? What can I do to protect myself from infection?"

& DISEASE TRANSMISSION

Herpes simplex II virus

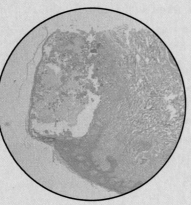

It is natural to have questions when helping in an emergency. Therefore it is important to know how diseases are transmitted and how to protect yourself when giving first aid.

Diseases that can pass from one person to another are called infectious diseases. Infectious diseases develop when germs invade the body and cause illness. The most common germs are bacteria and viruses.

Bacteria can live outside the body and do not depend on other organisms for life. The number of bacteria that infect humans is really very small. Some cause serious infections. These can be treated with special medications called antibiotics.

There are Some Simple Things You Can Do to Prevent Disease Transmission.

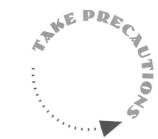

Viruses depend on other organisms to live. Once in the body, they are hard to remove. Few medications can fight viruses. The body's immune system is the number one protection against infection.

You may wonder how bacteria and viruses pass from one person to another. Well, in situations that require first aid care, diseases can be transmitted by touching, breathing, and biting.

You can become infected if you touch an infected person, if germs in that person's blood or other body fluids pass into your body through breaks or cuts in the skin or through the lining of your eyes, nose, and mouth. Therefore the greatest risk of infection occurs when you touch blood or other body fluids directly.

You can also be infected when you touch an object that has been soiled by a person's blood or body fluids. Be careful when handling soiled objects. Sharp objects can cut your skin and pass germs. Avoid touching blood and soiled objects with your bare hands.

Some diseases, such as the common cold, are transmitted by the air we breathe. It is possible to become infected if you breathe air exhaled by an infected person. Airborne infection can occur during sneezing, coughing, etc. Most of us are exposed to germs everyday in our jobs, on the bus, or in a crowded restaurant. Fortunately, simply being exposed to these germs is usually not adequate for diseases to be transmitted.

Animals can pass diseases through bites. For example, infected dogs, cats, cattle, and some wild animals can transmit rabies. A human bite also can pass disease. Contracting a disease from a bite is rare in any situation and very uncommon when giving first aid. In an emergency situation, it is unlikely that you will be bitten.

Some diseases are passed more easily than others. We all know how quickly the flu can pass from person to person at home or at work. Although these diseases can create discomfort, they are often temporary and are not serious to healthy adults.

Other diseases can be more serious, such as hepatitis B (HBV) and HIV, which causes AIDS. Although very serious, they are not easily transmitted and are not passed by casual contact, such as shaking hands. The primary way to transmit HBV or HIV is through blood-to-blood contact.
By following some basic guidelines, you can help reduce disease transmission when providing first aid:

- Avoid contact with body fluids when possible.
- Place barriers, such as disposable gloves or a clean dry cloth, between the victim's body fluids and yourself.
- Wear protective clothing, such as disposable gloves, to cover any cuts, scrapes, and skin conditions you may have.
- Wash your hands with soap and water immediately after giving care.
- Do not eat, drink, or touch your mouth, nose, or eyes when giving first aid.
- Do not touch objects that may be soiled with blood.
- Be prepared by having a first aid kit handy.

Following these guidelines decreases your risk of getting or transmitting an infectious disease. Remember always to give first aid in ways that protect you and the victim from disease transmission.

You Are More Likely to Give Care to a Family Member or a Friend Than to Someone You Do Not Know.

tion because of who the victim is. For example, the victim may be much older or much younger than you, be a different gender or race, have a disabling condition, be of a different status at work, or be a victim of a crime.

Sometimes people who have been injured or become suddenly ill act strangely or may be hard to deal with. The injury or illness, stress, or other factors such as the effects of drugs, alcohol, or medications may make people unpleasant or angry. Do not take this behavior personally. If you feel at all threatened by the victim's behavior, leave the immediate area and call your local emergency number for help.

Another factor that affects a person's decision to do something in an emergency is the type of injury or illness. An injury or illness may sometimes be very unpleasant. Blood, vomit, unpleasant odors, and deformed body parts or torn or burned skin upset almost everyone. You may have to turn away for a moment and take a few deep breaths to get control of your feelings. Then try to provide care. If you still cannot give first aid because of the way the injury looks, you can ensure your safety and the safety of victims and bystanders, and you can make sure you or someone else has called the local emergency number.

Disease transmission in a first aid situation is another issue that concerns many people. Nowadays, people worry about the possibility of catching a disease while giving first aid. This is especially true as a result of the AIDS epidemic. This concern is understandable. However, the actual risk of catching a disease when giving first aid is far less than you may think.

Giving first aid does not mean that you will automatically catch a disease. In fact, it is extremely unlikely that you will catch a disease by giving first aid. If you do not have any cuts or sores, your skin protects you as you give first aid. Remember that disease transmis-

sion works both ways. You can also pass diseases to the victim if you have any cuts or sores on your own skin.

Emergency situations that involve contact with body fluids, such as bleeding, have the possibility of transmitting disease. There are simple things you can do to minimize the chance of infection. Always take precautions to prevent direct contact with a victim's body fluids while you are giving first aid. When they are available, use protective barriers, such as disposable gloves or a clean cloth, to stop bleeding. The victim may even be able to use his or her own hand to help. Afterward, wash thoroughly as soon as possible, even if you wore gloves. Tell your doctor if you come in direct contact with a victim's body fluids while giving first aid.

Remember that you are most likely to use your first aid skills to help someone you know personally, such as a family member, friend, or co-worker. In some instances, you may know this person's health status and be aware of the risk of infection.

People react differently in emergencies. Whether trained in first aid or not, some people are afraid of doing the wrong thing and making matters worse. If you are not sure what to do, call your local emergency number for professional help. *The worst thing to do is nothing.*

Sometimes people worry that they might be sued for giving first aid. In fact, lawsuits against people who give emergency care at a scene of an accident are highly unusual and rarely successful. Most states have enacted "Good Samaritan" laws. These laws protect people who willingly give first aid without accepting anything in return. So you can help without worrying about lawsuits.

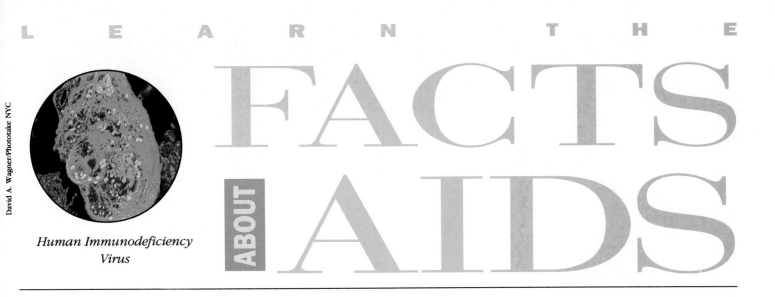

LEARN THE FACTS ABOUT AIDS

Human Immunodeficiency Virus

David A. Wagner/Phototake NYC

The Disease: AIDS stands for acquired immune deficiency syndrome. It is caused by the human immunodeficiency virus (HIV). When the virus gets into the body, it damages the immune system, the body system that fights infection. Once the virus enters the body, it can grow quietly in the body for months or even years. People infected with HIV might not feel or appear sick. Eventually, the weakened immune system gives way to certain types of infections.

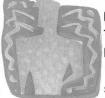

How the Disease is Transmitted: The virus enters the body in three basic ways:

■ Through direct contact with the bloodstream. *Example:* Sharing an unsterilized needle with an HIV-positive person to inject drugs into the veins.

■ Through the mucous membranes lining the eyes, mouth, throat, rectum, and vagina. *Example:* Having unprotected sex with an HIV-positive person—male or female.

■ Through the womb, birth canal, or breast milk. *Example:* Being infected as an unborn child or shortly after birth by an infected mother.

The virus cannot enter through the skin unless there is a cut or break in the skin. Even then, the possibility of infection is very low unless there is direct contact for a lengthy period of time. Saliva is not known to transmit HIV.

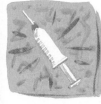

Prevention: Your behavior can put you at risk for getting AIDS. Using intravenous drugs, especially with unsterilized needles, or having sex without protection (such as condoms) are high-risk activities.

First Aid Precautions: The likelihood of HIV transmission during a first aid situation is very low. You are most likely to give first aid to someone you know, such as a family member or close friend. Always give care in ways that protect you and the victim from disease transmission. If possible, wash your hands before and after giving care, even if you wear disposable gloves. Avoid touching or being splashed by another person's body fluids, especially blood. Be prepared with a first aid kit that includes waterless antiseptic hand cleaners and disposable gloves.

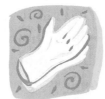

Testing: If you think you have put yourself at risk, get tested. A blood test will tell whether or not your body is producing antibodies in response to the virus.

If you are not sure whether you should be tested, call your doctor, the public health department, or the AIDS hot line listed below and talk to them. In the meantime, don't participate in activities that put anyone else at risk.

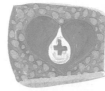

Blood Supply: Since 1985, all donated blood in the United States has been tested for HIV. As a result, the blood supply is considered safe. The risk of becoming infected through a blood transfusion is very low.

Hot Line: If you have questions, call the national AIDS hot line at 1-800-342-AIDS, 24 hours a day, 7 days a week, or the SIDA hot line (Spanish) at 1-800-344-SIDA, 8 a.m.-2 a.m., EST, 7 days a week. TTY/TDD service is available at 1-800-243-7TTY, Monday-Friday, 10 a.m.-10 p.m., EST, or call your state health department.

BE PREPARED

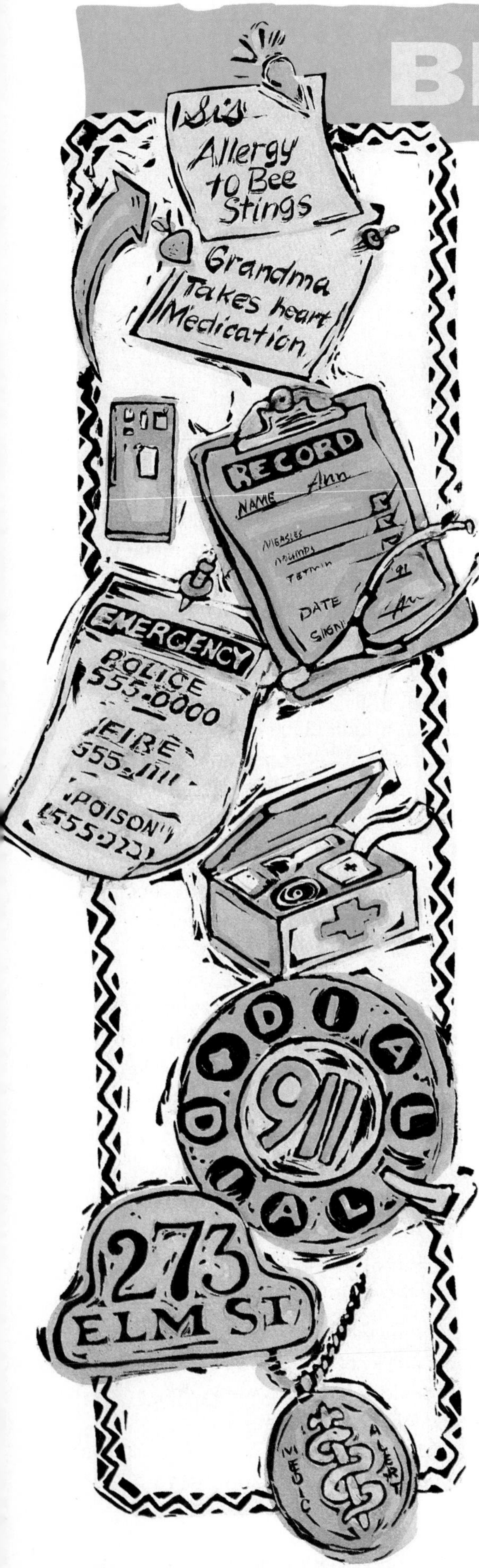

Keep information about you and your family in a handy place, such as on the refrigerator door or in your automobile glove compartment.

▼

Keep medical and insurance records up-to-date.

▼

Find out if your community is served by an emergency 9-1-1 telephone number. If it is not, look up the numbers for the police, fire department, EMS, and poison control center. Emergency numbers are usually listed in the front of the telephone book. Teach everyone in your home how and when to use these numbers.

▼

Keep emergency telephone numbers in a handy place, such as by the telephone or in the first aid kit. Include home and work numbers of family members and friends who can help. Be sure to keep both lists current.

▼

Keep a first aid kit handy in your home, automobile, workplace, and recreation area.

▼

Learn and practice first aid skills.

▼

Make sure your house or apartment number is easy to read. Numerals are easier to read than spelled-out numbers.

▼

Wear a medical alert tag if you have a potentially serious medical condition, such as epilepsy, diabetes, heart disease, or allergies.

Your decision to act in an emergency should be guided by your own values and by your knowledge of the risks that may be present. Your decision to act might not involve giving first aid. However, it should at least involve calling the local emergency number to get medical help.

PREPARING FOR EMERGENCIES

You will never see the emergencies you prevent. However, emergencies can and do happen, regardless of attempts to prevent them.

If you are prepared for unforeseen emergencies, you can help ensure that care begins as soon as possible—for yourself, your family, and your fellow citizens. If you are trained in first aid, you can give

help in the first few minutes of an emergency that can save a life. First aid *can* be the difference between life and death. Often it *does* make the difference between complete recovery and permanent disability.

By knowing what to do, you will be better able to manage your fears and overcome barriers to action. The most important things are to recognize that an emergency has occurred and to call the local emergency telephone number. Then give first aid until help arrives.

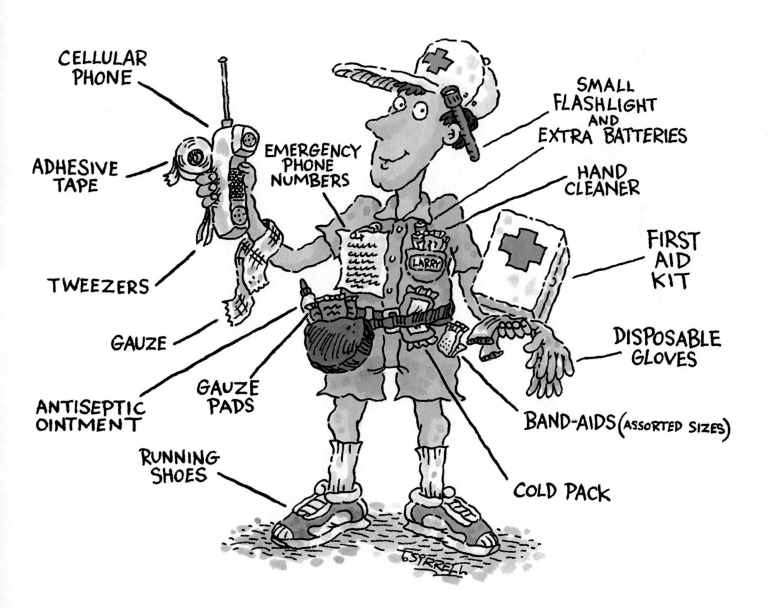

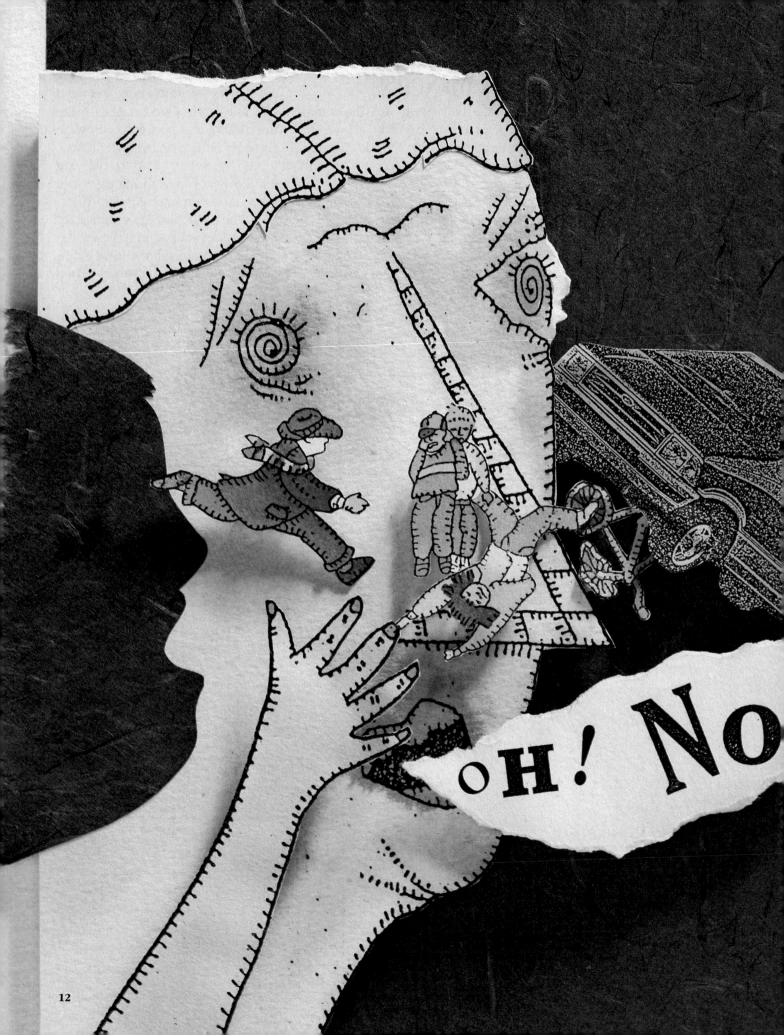

TAKING ACTION

It's 9:30 on a Saturday morning. The sudden sounds outside are close together but very clear—a screech of brakes, a thud, and a shrill scream. You are out the door and onto the sidewalk before you have time to think about it. Maria and Rose had been playing out there!

People are running from all over. Your eyes take it in—the twisted bike, the van in the middle of the street, and the child lying on the pavement. At least he's alive; he's moaning and crying. His left leg looks funny and there's blood on the pavement. A man is staring at the boy. "He just came out of nowhere," he stammers. "All of a sudden, there he was, right in front of the van." The boy is obviously hurt. What should you do?

So far, you've learned that you can make a difference in an emergency. You may even save a life. You now know how to recognize an emergency. You've learned that the worst thing you can do is nothing and deciding to get involved can be hard for anyone—not just you. You also know some things you can do to help.

Even so, when an emergency happens, you may feel confused. However, you can train yourself to stay calm and think before you act. Ask yourself, "What do I need to do? What is the best help I can give?" To answer these questions, you should know three basic steps you can take in any emergency:

1. *Check* the scene and the victim.
2. *Call* 9-1-1 or your local emergency number.
3. *Care* for the victim.

CHECK

Before you can help the victim, you must make sure the scene is safe for you and any bystanders. You also need some information.

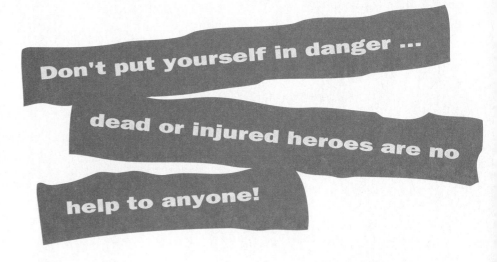

Look the scene over and try to answer these questions:

1. Is the scene safe?
2. What happened?
3. How many victims are there?
4. Can bystanders help?

Check for anything that might make the scene unsafe. Examples include spilled chemicals, traffic, fire, escaping steam, downed electrical lines, smoke, extreme weather, and poisonous gas. If these or other dangers threaten, do not go near the victim. Stay at a safe distance and call your local emergency number immediately.

If the scene is still unsafe after you call, stay away from the victim. Don't put yourself in danger. Dead or injured heroes are no help to anyone! Leave dangerous situations to professionals like fire fighters and police who have the training and equipment to deal with them. Once they make the scene safe, you can offer to help.

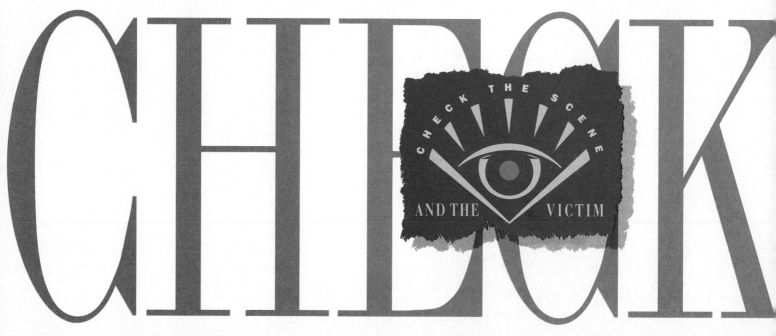

Try to find out what happened. Look for clues to what caused the emergency and how the victim might be injured. Nearby objects, such as a fallen ladder, broken glass, or a spilled bottle of medicine, may give you information. Your check of the scene may be the only way to tell what happened.

Look carefully for more than one victim. You might not spot everyone at first. If one victim is bleeding or screaming, you might not notice an unconscious victim. It is also easy to overlook a baby or a small child. Once you reach the victim, check the scene again. You may see dangers, clues, or victims you missed before.

Do not move a seriously injured victim unless there is an immediate danger, such as fire, flood, or poisonous gas. If you must move the victim, do it as quickly and carefully as possible. If there is no danger, tell the victim not to move. Tell any bystanders not to move the victim.

You have already learned that the presence of bystanders does not mean that a victim is receiving help. Besides doing what you can for the victim, you can ask bystanders to help. They may be able to tell you what happened or direct you to the nearest telephone. A family member, friend, or co-worker who is present may know if the victim has an illness or a medical condition. The victim may be too upset to answer your questions. A child may be especially frightened. This may also be true for an adult who has been unconscious for a few minutes. Bystanders can also help comfort the victim and others at the scene. Parents or guardians who are present may be able to calm a frightened child. They can also tell you if a child has a medical condition.

When you reach the victim, you must try to find out what is wrong. Look for signals that may indicate a life-threatening emergency. The first thing you check is whether the victim is conscious. Sometimes this is obvious. The victim may be able to speak to you and tell you what happened. The victim may be moaning, crying, or making some other noise. The victim may be moving around. Talk to the victim to reassure him or her and to learn what you can about what happened.

What if the victim is lying on the ground, silent, and not moving? You must find out if the victim is conscious or unconscious. Unconsciousness is a life-threatening emergency. If the victim doesn't respond to you in any way, assume he or she is unconscious. You must call for an ambulance at once!

Look for other signals of injuries that are life-threatening or may become life-threatening: no breathing or breathing with difficulty, no pulse, and/or severe bleeding.

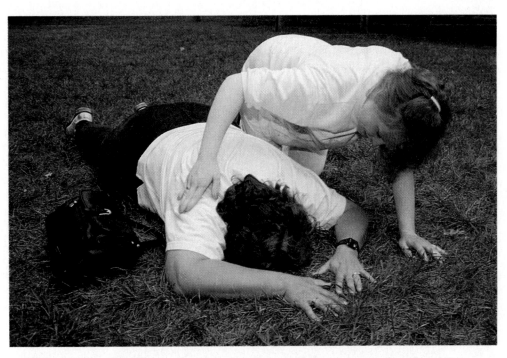

If the victim doesn't respond to you in any way, assume the victim is unconscious. Call for an ambulance at once!

"Do No Further Harm"

One of the most dangerous threats to a seriously injured victim is unnecessary movement. Usually when giving care, you will not face dangers that require you to move a victim. In most cases, you can follow the emergency steps (check, call, and care) where you find the victim. Moving the victim can cause additional injury and pain and complicate the victim's recovery.

There are three general situations in which you should move a victim. The most obvious is when you are faced with immediate danger such as fire, lack of oxygen, risk of explosion, or a collapsing structure.

A second reason to move a victim is if you have to get to another victim who may have a more serious problem. In this case, you may have to move a victim with minor injuries to reach one who needs care immediately. Third, you may have to move the victim to provide proper care. For example, someone who has collapsed and does not have a pulse needs cardiopulmonary resuscitation (CPR). CPR needs to be performed on a firm, flat surface. If the surface or space is not adequate to provide care, the victim should be moved.

Once you decide to move a victim, you must quickly decide *how* to move the victim. Carefully consider your safety and the safety of the victim. Base your decision on the dangers you are facing, the size and condition of the victim, your ability and condition, and whether you have any help.

You can improve your chances of successfully moving a victim without injuring yourself. When you lift, use your legs, not your back. Bend your body at the knees and hips and avoid twisting your body. Walk forward when possible, taking small steps, and looking where you are going.

Avoid twisting or bending the victim with a possible head or spine injury. Do not move a victim who is too large to move comfortably.

You can help support a victim who is conscious and who can walk with assistance. Place the victim's arm over your shoulders and hold it in place with your hand. Support the victim with your other arm around the victim's waist. If you have another person to help you, he or she can support the victim the same way on the other side.

If you have a second rescuer to help, you can also carry a victim who can't walk. The seat carry provides a secure way for two people to carry a victim. The two rescuers face each other

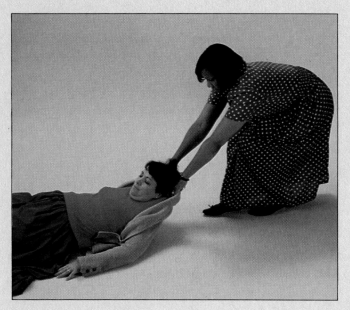

The clothes drag.

and interlock their arms, each with one arm under the victim's thighs and one arm behind the victim's back. The victim is lifted by the seat formed by the rescuers' arms.

If you are alone and the victim can't walk with assistance, you can drag the victim. Use the victim's clothes (e.g., shirt, coat, or sweater) to drag the victim if you suspect a head or spine injury. Gather the victim's clothes tightly behind the victim's neck. Use the clothes to pull the victim. Support the head with the clothes and your hands.

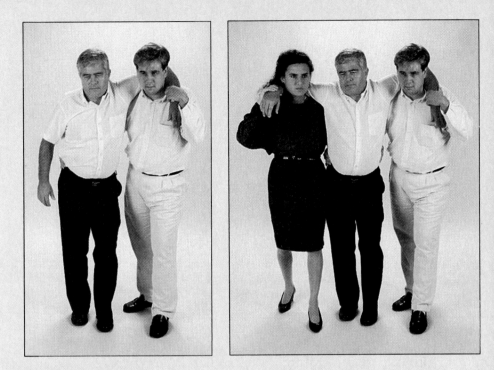

The walking assist.

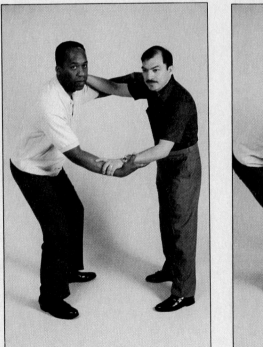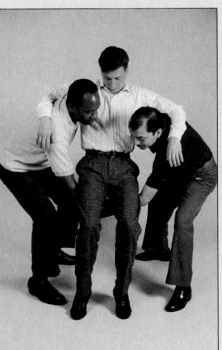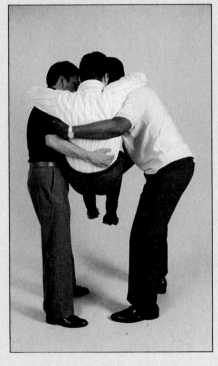

The two-person seat carry.

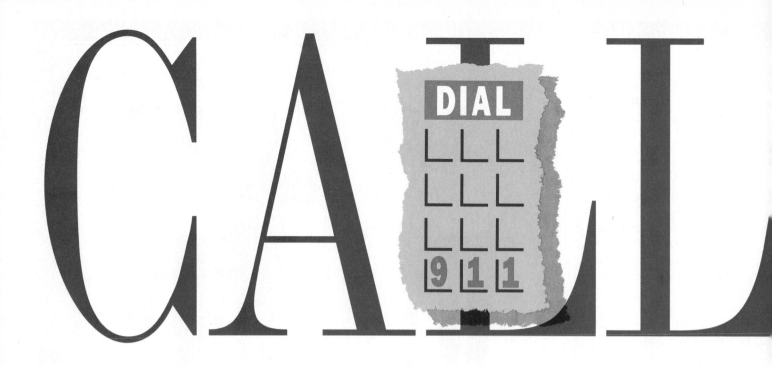

CALL

While you are checking the victim, use your senses of sight, smell, and hearing. They will help you notice anything abnormal. For example, an unusual smell may be caused by a poison. You may see a bruise or a twisted arm or leg. Listen carefully to what the victim says.

CALL

It is very important that you know your local emergency number. It may be 9-1-1, 0 for operator, a local seven-digit number, or a special response number where you work. Post your emergency number by the phone at home and at work.

Calling for help is often the most important action you can take to help the victim! It will start professional emergency help on its way as fast as possible. Whenever possible, ask a bystander to make the call for you. When possible, tell the caller the victim's condition so that he or she can tell the dispatcher. Tell the caller not to hang up before the dispatcher does. This might cut off some information the

dispatcher needs to have or give. There is no hard, fast rule of when to call your emergency number.

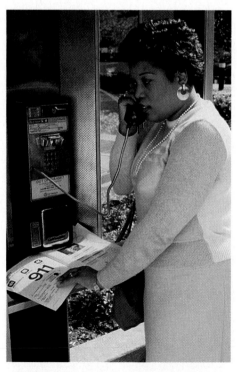

Calling for help is often the most important action you can take to help the victim.

You have to use your own judgment. *In general, the best guideline is: when in doubt . . . call.*

If you are the only person on the scene, shout for help. If the victim is unconscious and no one comes at once to help you, you will need to get professional help fast. Find the nearest telephone as quickly as possible. Make the call and go back to the victim. Recheck the victim and give the necessary care.

If you shout and no one responds while you are giving urgent care, such as controlling severe bleeding, continue for about a minute while you think where to find the nearest telephone. Then get to that telephone as quickly as possible. After making the call, return to the victim.

It is clear that you should call your local emergency number if a victim is unconscious. You should also call if a victim is faint, drowsy, confused, dizzy, or drifts in and out of consciousness.

Call for an ambulance if a victim is having trouble breathing or is breathing in an unnatural way. A victim who is breathing very slowly, heavily, or rapidly, or gasping for breath might not be getting enough air or may stop breathing. A victim who is making rasping, shrill, gurgling, or choking noises may be in similar danger. A victim who has no pulse does not have a beating heart. A victim who is bleeding severely will die after losing a large amount of blood. These are life-threatening conditions requiring the rapid assistance of medical professionals.

Other conditions may be less obvious but no less dangerous. A victim with pain or pressure in the chest or abdomen may well have injuries you can't see—internal injuries—and so may the victim who is vomiting or passing blood.

Seizures, a severe headache, and slurred speech can all be signals of serious injury. The victim may be poisoned, have a head or spinal injury, or have some other dangerous condition, so call. If you suspect the victim has one or more broken bones, call for an ambulance also. If not cared for properly, fractures can cause both immediate and long-term problems.

You also need to call 9-1-1 or your local emergency number for certain situations that must be dealt with only by trained and equipped people. Fire and explosion are situations of this type and so are downed electrical wires and swiftly moving or rapidly rising water. They make a scene unsafe, and you must always stay at a safe distance when any of these conditions are part of an emergency scene.

Poisonous gas can be harder to detect. Sometimes it has no odor or color. You might suspect poisonous gas is present if you see people who are unconscious or behaving strangely for no apparent reason. Call your emergency number. Call also for vehicle collisions and for situations in which victims cannot

When To Call

EMS

If the victim is unconscious, call 9-1-1 or your local emergency number immediately. Sometimes a conscious victim will tell you not to call an ambulance, and you may not be sure what to do. Call for an ambulance anyway if the victim —

Is or becomes unconscious.

Has trouble breathing or is breathing in a strange way.

Has chest pain or pressure.

Is bleeding severely.

Has pressure or pain in the abdomen that does not go away.

Is vomiting or passing blood.

Has seizures, a severe headache, or slurred speech.

Appears to have been poisoned.

Has injuries to the head, neck, or back.

Has possible broken bones.

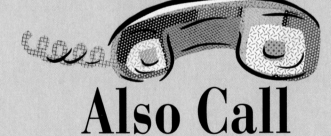

Also Call

Also call for any of these situations:

Fire or explosion

Downed electrical wires

Swiftly moving or rapidly rising water

Presence of poisonous gas

Vehicle collisions

Victims who cannot be moved easily

HOW TO CALL EMS

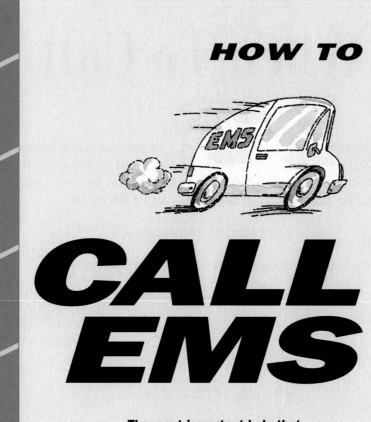

The most important help that you can provide to a victim who is unconscious or has some other life-threatening emergency is to call for professional medical help. Make the call quickly and return to the victim. If possible, send someone else to make the call. Be sure that you or another caller follows these four steps:

1 Call the emergency number. The number is 9-1-1 in many communities. In others, it is a seven-digit number. Dial 0 (the operator) if you do not know the number in the area.

2 Give the dispatcher the necessary information. Answer any questions that he or she might ask. Most dispatchers will ask:

- The exact location or address of the emergency. Include the name of the city or town, nearby intersections, landmarks, the building name, the floor, and the room or apartment number.
- The telephone number from which the call is being made.
- The caller's name.
- What happened — for example, a motor vehicle collision, fire, or fall.
- How many people are involved.
- The condition of the victim(s) — for example, unconsciousness, chest pains, or severe bleeding.
- What help (first aid) is being given.

3 Do not hang up until the dispatcher hangs up. The EMS dispatcher may be able to tell you how to best care for the victim.

4 Return and continue to care for the victim.

With a life-threatening emergency, the survival of a victim often depends on both professional medical help *and* the care you can provide. You will have to use your best judgment, based on knowledge of your surroundings, knowledge gained from this course, and other training you may have received to make the decision to call. Generally, *call FAST!*

WHAT HAPPENS WHEN YOU CALL EMS

When your call is answered, you will be talking to an emergency dispatcher who has had special training in dealing with crises over the phone.

The dispatcher will ask you for your phone number and address and will ask other key questions to determine whether you need police, fire, or medical assistance.

It may seem that the dispatcher asks a lot of questions. The information you give will help the dispatcher to send the type of help you need, based on the severity of the emergency.

Once the ambulance is on the way, the dispatcher may stay on the line and continue to talk with you. Many dispatchers today are also trained to give instructions before EMS arrival, so they can assist you with certain life-saving techniques, such as CPR or rescue breathing, until the ambulance arrives.

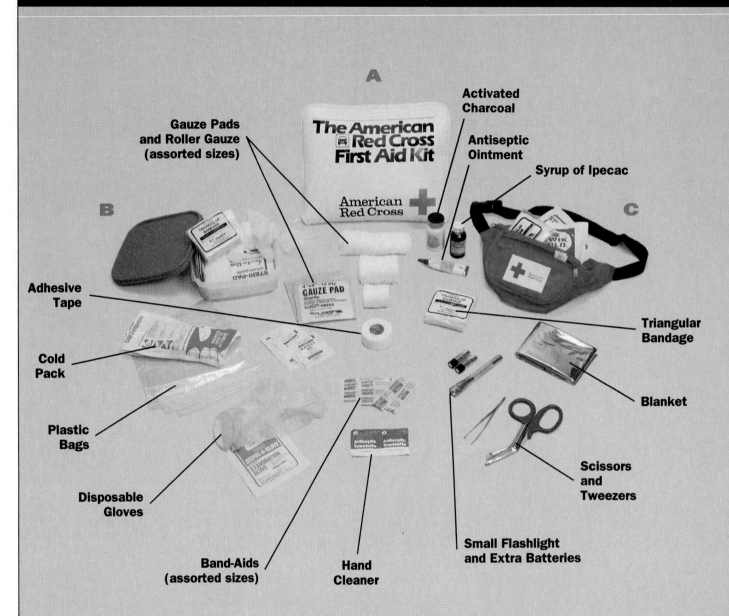

A

Activated Charcoal

Gauze Pads and Roller Gauze (assorted sizes)

The American Red Cross First Aid Kit

American Red Cross

Antiseptic Ointment

Syrup of Ipecac

B

C

Adhesive Tape

GAUZE PAD Sterile

Triangular Bandage

Cold Pack

Blanket

Plastic Bags

Scissors and Tweezers

Disposable Gloves

Band-Aids (assorted sizes)

Hand Cleaner

Small Flashlight and Extra Batteries

A well-stocked first aid kit is a handy thing to have. To be prepared for emergencies, keep a first aid kit in your home and in your automobile. Carry a first aid kit with you or know where you can find one when you are hiking, biking, camping, or boating. Find out the location of first aid kits where you work.

First aid kits come in many shapes and sizes. **A**, You can buy one from a drug store, or your local Red Cross chapter may sell them. **B**, You can make your own first aid kit. **C**, Some kits are designed for specific activities, such as hiking, camping, or boating. Whether you buy a first aid kit or put one together, make sure it has all the items you may need. Include any personal items, such as medications and emergency phone numbers, or other items your physician may suggest. Check the kit regularly. Make sure the flashlight batteries work. Check expiration dates and replace any used or out-of-date contents.

be reached or moved easily. They may be trapped in cars or in buildings, for example. Call also for emergencies involving more than one victim.

These circumstances aren't a complete list. There are always exceptions. Trust your instincts. If you think there is an emergency, there probably is. If you are confused or unsure about what care to give, call for an ambulance at once. EMS personnel would rather come and find no emergency than arrive at an emergency too late to help.

CARE

Once you have checked the scene and the victim, you may need to provide care. To do this, you can follow some general steps of care. Always care for life-threatening emergencies before those that are not life-threatening. While you are waiting for the ambulance, watch for changes in the victim's breathing and consciousness. Help the victim rest comfortably. Keep him or her from getting chilled or overheated. Reassure the victim.

If the victim is conscious and able to talk, he or she is breathing and has a pulse. Introduce yourself, ask the victim's permission for you to help. Ask what happened and if the victim hurts anywhere. If the victim has pain, ask where the pain is located and what it is like— burning, aching, sharp, stinging. Ask when it started and how bad it

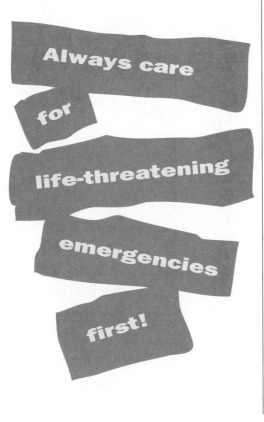

Always care for life-threatening emergencies first!

Getting Permission to Give Care

You may want to care for an injured or ill person, but before giving first aid, you must have the victim's permission. To get permission you *must* tell the victim who you are, how much training you have, and how you plan to help. Only then can a conscious victim give you permission to give care.

Do not give care to a conscious victim who refuses it. If the conscious victim is an infant or child, permission to give care should be obtained from a supervising adult when one is available. If the condition is serious, permission is implied if a supervising adult is not present.

Permission is also implied if a victim is unconscious or unable to respond. This means that you can assume that, if the person could respond, he or she would agree to care.

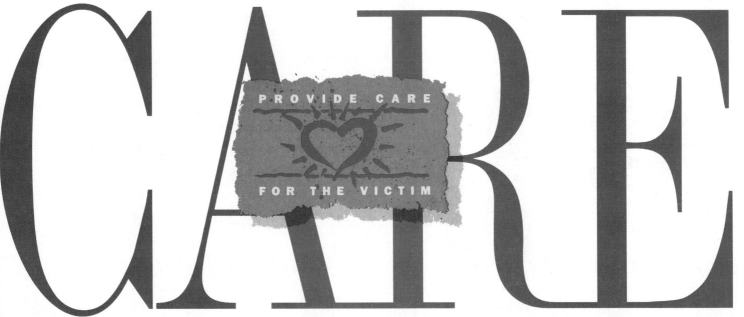

PROVIDE CARE FOR THE VICTIM

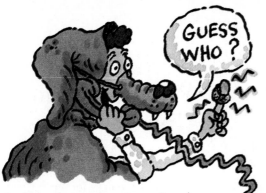

is. Be calm and patient. Speak normally and simply.

After you have finished checking the victim and giving care, you might decide it is OK to take the victim to a hospital or doctor yourself. Be very careful about making this decision. Do not transport a victim with a life-threatening condition or one that could become life-threatening.

A car trip can be painful for the victim. It can also make an injury worse. If you do decide to transport the victim, always have someone else come with you. Watch the victim carefully for any changes in condition. Be sure you know the fastest route. **Do not let the victim drive, either alone or with you.**

When you respond to an emergency, remember the emergency action steps: check, call, and care. They guide your actions in an emergency and ensure your safety and the safety of others. By following these steps, you can give the victim of a serious illness or injury the best chance of survival.

Don't Cry Wolf!

Your local emergency number is for just that—emergencies! It should not be misused. Nonemergency calls account for about 30 to 40 percent of all 9-1-1 calls in many U.S. cities. So please, use good judgment.

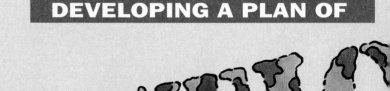

DEVELOPING A PLAN OF

ACTIO

Emergencies can happen quickly. There may be no time to think about what you should do. There may be only enough time to react. You can improve your reaction and change the outcome of the emergency by planning.

Everyone has a plan of action. It may be instinct. It may be as simple as, "I'm scared . . . run!" Running may even work—if you can run fast enough and in the right direction. Most of us do not want to base how well we deal with emergencies on how fast we run. We would rather find a way to improve our chances. We need a well–thought-out plan.

A good plan identifies the emergencies you are most likely to face. The plan also identifies the possible location and the persons involved. All of this information can help you to define the size and scope of a possible emergency. Now, you can begin to decide how you would respond and what other information and training you would need.

The first step in planning is to gather information. Here are some suggestions on where to start.

First, think about your home.
- Type of home (mobile, high rise, duplex, single family, etc.)
- Type of construction (wood, brick, etc.)
- Location of sleeping areas

- Number and location of smoke alarms
- Location of gasoline, solvent, or paint storage
- Number and types of locks on doors
- Location of telephones
- Location of flashlights
- Location of fire extinguisher
- Location of first aid kit

Think about who lives there.
- Number of people living in the home
- Number of people over 65 or under 6 years of age
- Number of people sleeping above or below the ground floor
- Number of people unable to exit without help

Think about the types of emergencies that you may face at home.
- Injuries (like a fall or a cut)
- Illnesses (like a stroke or a heart attack)
- Natural disasters (like a tornado or an earthquake)
- Fire

Now that you have information, you can start to plan.
Get help from the people you live with. Write the list of emergencies and under each emergency, list —
1. The way the emergency would affect your home.
2. The way you would like the people in your home to react.
3. The steps you have taken to prevent or minimize the effect of the emergency.
4. The steps you need to take.

For example, when discussing fire you might list —
1. The fire could burn all or part of our home.
2. If the fire started on the stove while someone was cooking, that person should use a fire extinguisher to put out the fire. If the fire could not be controlled, he or she should call the emergency number, have everyone leave the house, and leave also. Then everyone should meet at the tree in the front yard.
3. Smoke alarms are in the kitchen, the stairwells, and outside the bedrooms. A fire extinguisher is in the kitchen.
4. We should make sure the fire extinguisher is charged and everyone should know how to operate it. We should also make sure everyone knows what to do.

If you need more help, here are other sources of information:
- Insurance companies
- Your city or county Emergency Management office
- Your police department
- Your fire department/rescue squad

Try to imagine as many situations as possible for each emergency. Think about emergencies away from home. Use the same process to decide what to do. When people have questions, others living in the home can help decide what action to take.

When you reach a decision, write it down. You now have a personal plan. Practice it. Keep it current.

FIRST AID CHALLENGE

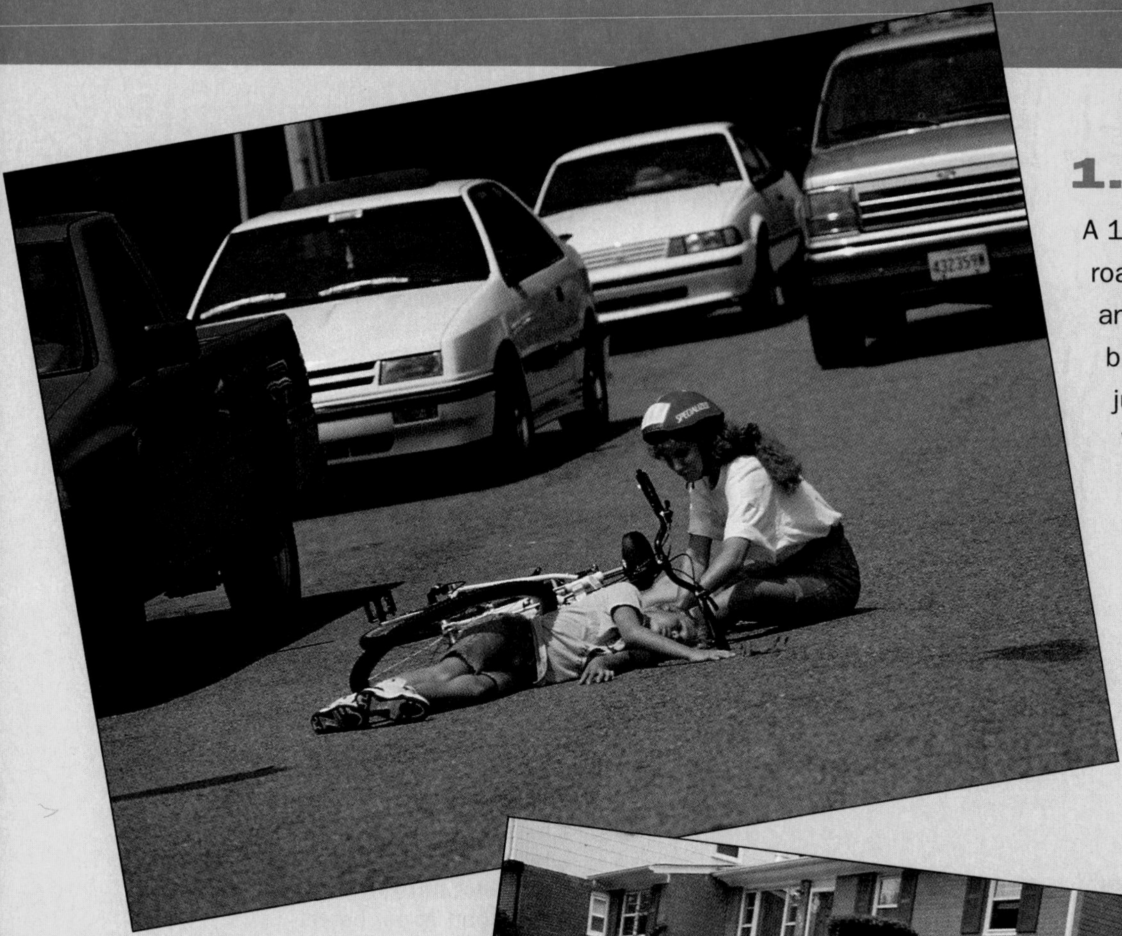

1.

A 10-year-old child darts onto the road between two parked cars and is struck by an oncoming bicyclist. Both victims are injured on the busy road.
What would you do?

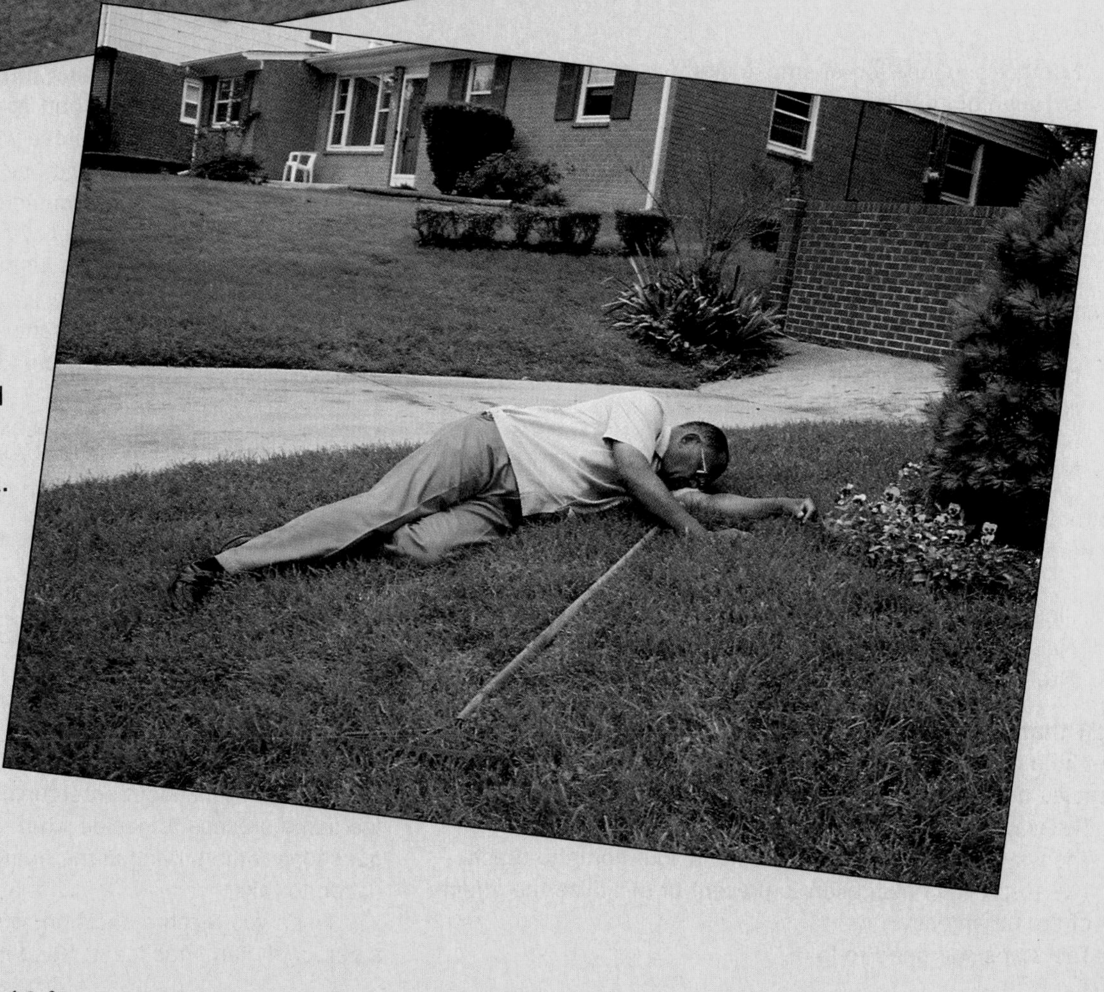

2.

You witness your 60-year-old neighbor grasp his chest and suddenly collapse on the ground while doing yard work. He does not appear to be breathing. What would you do?

You have learned the emergency action steps that can be applied in any emergency—check, call, and care. Would you know what to do in an emergency? Test your knowledge of the emergency action steps by deciding what you would do in each of the four situations below. If you are unsure how you should proceed in any of the four situations, review the information in the "Taking Action" article.

3.

Your 50-year-old relative has been complaining of an "unusual tightness" in her chest and nausea for several hours. Suddenly she experiences severe pain in her chest and is now having trouble breathing. What would you do?

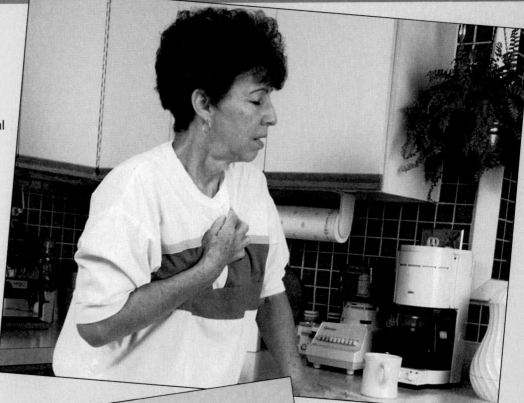

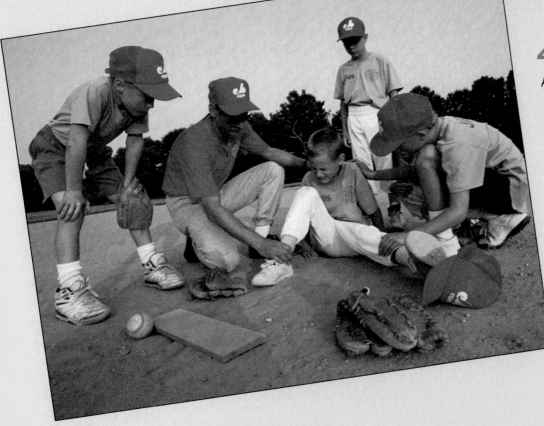

4.

A pitcher on a little league baseball team has been struck in the ankle by a line-drive. He falls to the ground in pain and is unable to move his foot. What would you do?

CHECKING

When you reach the victim, check first for life-threatening conditions, such as unconsciousness. In many emergencies, you will know right away whether the victim is unconscious. However, in some situations, you may not be able to tell. If you are not sure whether a victim is unconscious, tap the victim on one shoulder.

Always begin by determining if a victim is conscious. To find out if a victim is conscious, tap him or her on one shoulder. Ask the victim if he or she is OK. If you know the person, use his or her name. Speak loudly. If the victim does not respond to you, assume he or she is unconscious. Call for an ambulance at once.

THE VICTIM

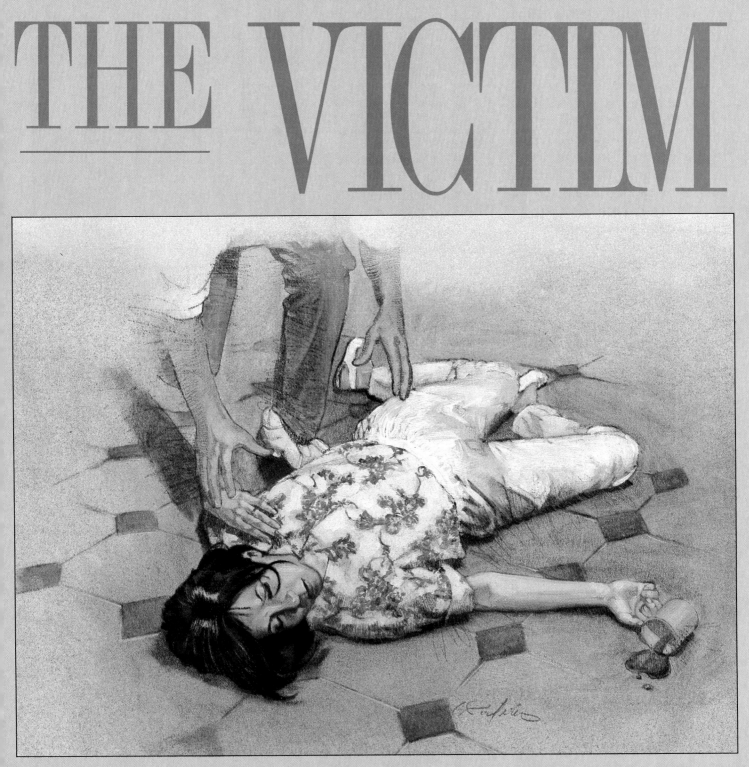

CHECKING AN UNCONSCIOUS VICTIM

After you call for an ambulance, you should return immediately to the victim. If you send another person to call, check the victim while the other person is calling. You must find out if there are other conditions that threaten the victim's life. You should check to see if an unconscious victim—

• Is breathing.
• Has a pulse.
• Is bleeding severely.

If the victim is not breathing, the victim's life is threatened. To check to see if the victim is breathing, put your head near the victim's mouth and nose. Look, listen, and feel for breathing for about 5 seconds. At the same time, watch the chest to see if it rises and falls.

Perhaps the victim isn't in a position where you can do this. For example, the victim may be facedown, and you can't tell whether

If the victim does not respond to you, assume he or she is unconscious. Call for an ambulance at once!

Check to see if an unconscious victim—

- **Is Breathing.**
- **Has a Pulse.**
- **Is Bleeding Severely.**

the victim is breathing. In this case, roll the victim gently onto his or her back. Be sure to keep the head and back in as straight a line as possible while you roll the victim.

Tip the victim's head back and lift the chin, then recheck breathing. If the victim is breathing, the victim's heart is beating and circulating blood. If the victim is not breathing, you must immediately give the victim a couple of breaths. Then find out if the victim's heart is beating by checking the pulse.

To check the pulse in an adult or a child, feel at the front of the neck for the Adam's apple and slide your fingers into the groove next to it in the side of the neck. If the heart is beating, you will feel the

beat of the blood in one of the big blood vessels that run along both sides of the neck. With a baby, feel in the arm midway between the elbow and the shoulder. This beat you feel in the neck or the arm is called the pulse. Take about 5 seconds to feel for the pulse.

If the victim has a pulse but is still not breathing, you will have to do rescue breathing. If the victim does not have a pulse, the heart is not beating properly. You must keep blood circulating in the victim's body until medical help arrives. To do this, you will have to give cardiopulmonary resuscitation (CPR). Rescue breathing and CPR are discussed in a later article called "When Seconds Count."

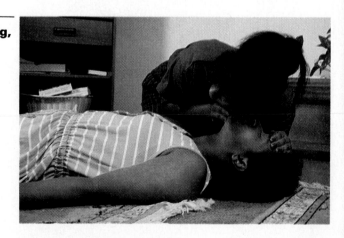

To check for breathing, look, listen, and feel for breathing. Watch the chest to see if it rises.

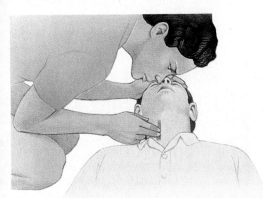

To find out if the heart is beating, check the pulse. Check the pulse of an adult or child at the side of the neck. Check the pulse of an infant at the inside of the arm between the shoulder and the elbow.

Adult

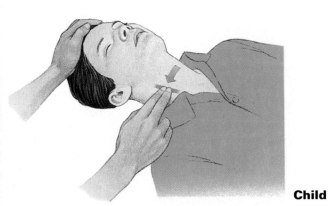

Child

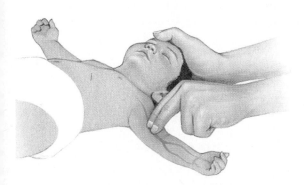

Infant

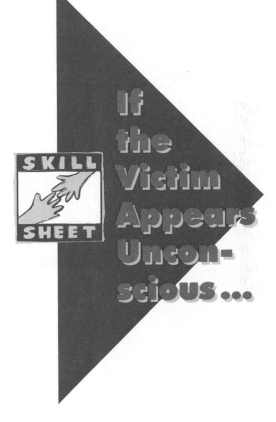

If the Victim Appears Unconscious...

SKILL SHEET

Check for bleeding by looking over the victim's body from head to toe for signs of bleeding such as blood-soaked clothing. Bleeding is severe, for example, when blood spurts out of a wound. Bleeding usually looks worse than it is. A small amount of blood on a slick surface or mixed with water almost always looks like a great deal of blood. It isn't always easy to recognize severe bleeding. You will have to make a decision based on your best judgment. If you think bleed- ing is severe, call your local emergency number.

CHECKING A CONSCIOUS VICTIM

If the victim is conscious, ask what happened. If the victim is able to speak with you, he or she is breathing and has a pulse. Look for other life-threatening conditions and conditions that need care or might become life-threatening. The victim may be able to tell you what

Check the Victim

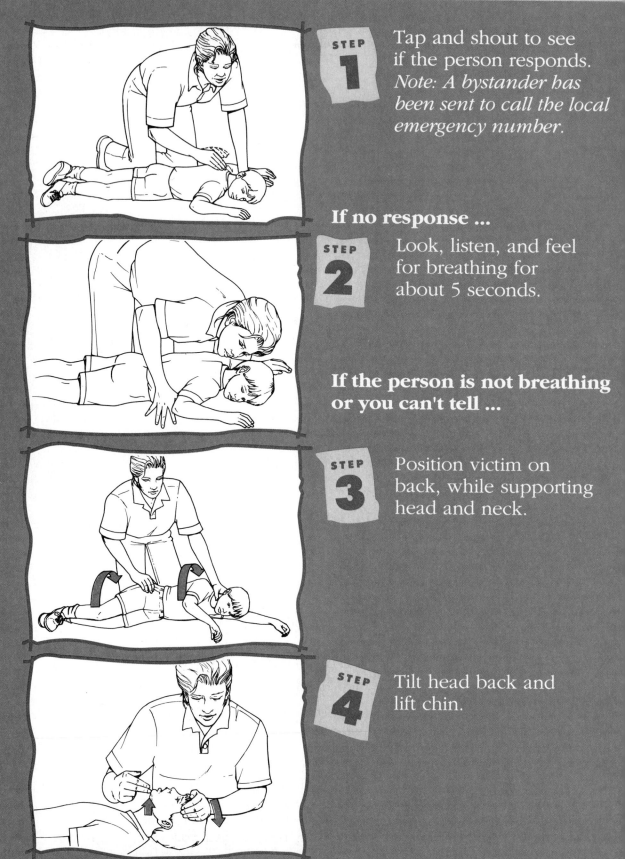

STEP 1

Tap and shout to see if the person responds. *Note: A bystander has been sent to call the local emergency number.*

If no response ...

STEP 2

Look, listen, and feel for breathing for about 5 seconds.

If the person is not breathing or you can't tell ...

STEP 3

Position victim on back, while supporting head and neck.

STEP 4

Tilt head back and lift chin.

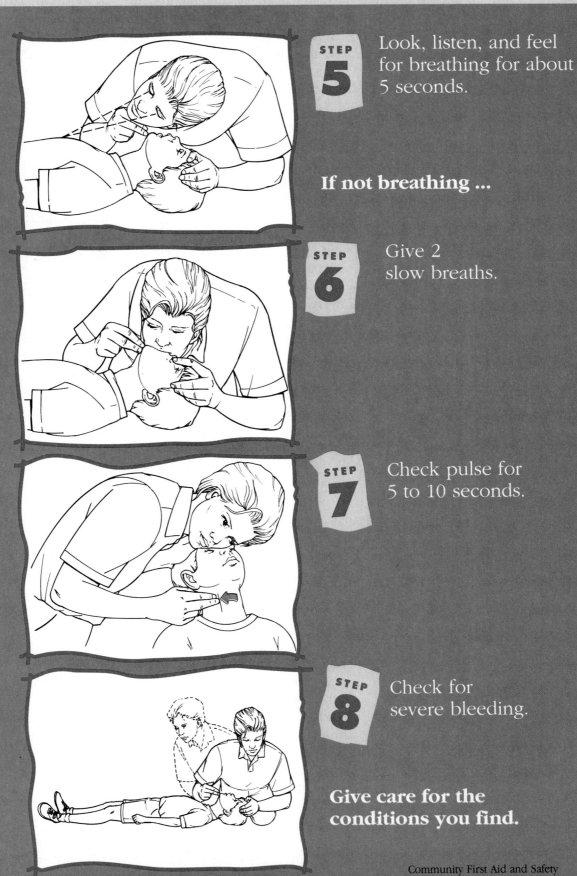

STEP 5 Look, listen, and feel for breathing for about 5 seconds.

If not breathing ...

STEP 6 Give 2 slow breaths.

STEP 7 Check pulse for 5 to 10 seconds.

STEP 8 Check for severe bleeding.

Give care for the conditions you find.

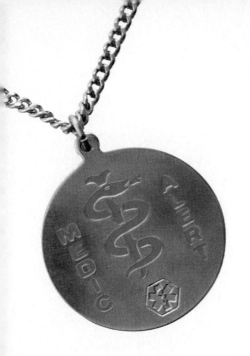

Medical alert tags can provide important medical information about the victim.

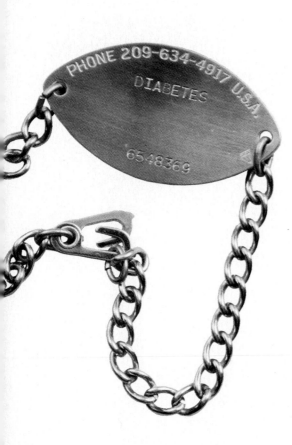

happened and how he or she feels. This information helps determine what care may be needed.

This check has two steps:

1. Talk to the victim and to any people standing by who saw the emergency take place.
2. Check the victim from head to toe, so you do not overlook any problems.

Don't ask the victim to move, and do not move the victim yourself. Injured people will find the most comfortable position to be in.

Begin your check at the victim's head, examining the scalp, face, ears, nose, and mouth. Look for cuts, bruises, bumps, or depressions. Watch for changes in consciousness. Notice if the victim is drowsy, not alert, or confused. Look for changes in the victim's breathing. A healthy person breathes regularly, quietly, and easily. Babies and young children normally breathe faster than adults. Breathing that is not normal includes noisy breathing such as gasping for air; making rasping, gurgling, or whistling sounds; breathing unusually fast or slow; and breathing that is painful.

Notice how the skin looks and feels. Note if the skin is reddish, bluish, pale, or gray. Feel with the back of your hand on the forehead to see if the skin feels unusually damp, dry, cool, or hot. The skin can provide clues that the victim is injured or sick.

Look over the body. Ask again about any areas that hurt. Ask the victim to move each part of the body that doesn't hurt. Check the shoulders by asking the victim to shrug them. Check the chest and abdomen by asking the victim to take a deep breath. Ask the victim if he or she can move the fingers,

hands, and arms. Check the hips and legs in the same way. *During a head-to-toe check, don't touch any painful areas; don't ask the victim to move any parts that hurt.* Watch the victim's face for signs of pain and listen for sounds of pain such as gasps, moans, or cries.

Look for odd bumps or depressions. Think of how the body usually looks. If you are not sure if

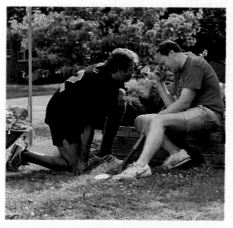

If a victim is able to talk, you know he or she is breathing and has a pulse.

something is out of shape, check it against the other side of the body.

Look for a medical alert tag on the victim's wrist or neck. A tag will give you medical information about the victim, care to give for that problem, and whom to call for help.

When you have finished checking, if the victim can move his or her body without any pain and there are no other signs of injury, have the victim rest sitting up. When the victim feels ready, help him or her stand up.

As you continue reading, you will learn more about life-threatening emergencies, such as breathing and heart problems.

Changing everyday habits can improve the quality of your life and reduce the possibility of illness and injury. The following list of statements can help you to identify some important steps toward a healthier and safer life. Mark each box next to the statement that represents your actions. Unmarked boxes identify areas that put you at risk.

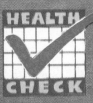

HEALTHY LIFE-STYLE IQ QUIZ

Stress
- [ ] 1. I plan my days off to allow time for recreation.
- [ ] 2. I get enough sleep.
- [ ] 3. I express feelings of anger and worry.
- [ ] 4. I make decisions with little or no worry.
- [ ] 5. I set realistic goals for myself.
- [ ] 6. I accept responsibility for my actions.
- [ ] 7. I manage stress so that it does not affect my physical well-being.
- [ ] 8. I discuss problems with friends and relatives.

Physical Health
- [ ] 9. I eat a balanced diet.
- [ ] 10. I have regular medical check-ups.
- [ ] 11. I have regular dental check-ups.
- [ ] 12. I have regular eye examinations.
- [ ] 13. I avoid using illegal substances.
- [ ] 14. I have fewer than five alcoholic beverages per week.
- [ ] 15. I avoid using alcoholic beverages when taking medications.
- [ ] 16. When taking medications, I follow the directions on the label.

Personal Safety
- [ ] 17. I keep my vehicle in good operating condition.
- [ ] 18. I obey traffic laws.
- [ ] 19. I wear safety belts whenever I operate my automobile.
- [ ] 20. I keep recreational equipment in good working condition.
- [ ] 21. I wear life jackets (personal flotation devices – PFDs) when taking part in water activities, such as boating, fishing, and waterskiing.
- [ ] 22. I swim only when others are present.

Home Safety
- [ ] 23. I post local emergency number(s) near my telephone(s).
- [ ] 24. I have battery-operated smoke detectors where I live.
- [ ] 25. I keep medications safely and securely stored out of the reach of children.
- [ ] 26. I keep cleansers and other poisonous materials safely and securely stored.
- [ ] 27. I turn off the oven and other appliances after use.
- [ ] 28. I keep a working fire extinguisher in my home.
- [ ] 29. I have an emergency plan in the event of injury, sudden illness, or natural disaster.
- [ ] 30. I practice emergency plans with my family or roommates.

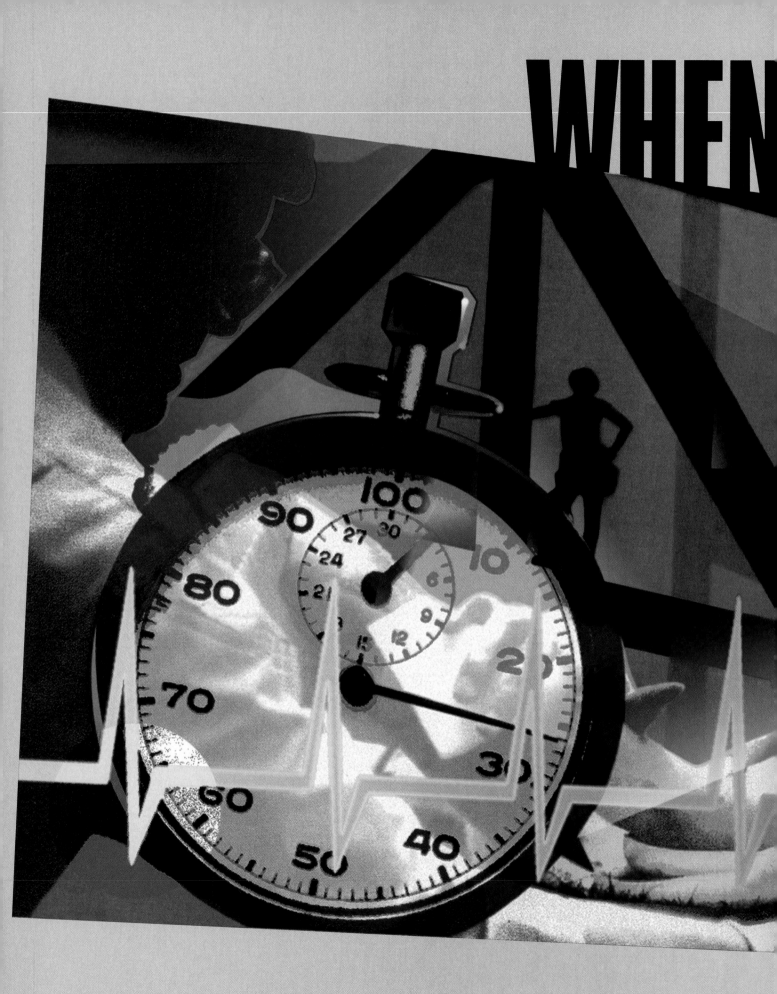

WHEN

SECONDS COUNT

In a life-threatening emergency, you must help at once. It may only be a matter of seconds before the person dies. An emergency is life-threatening if the victim is unconscious, is not breathing, is breathing with difficulty, has no pulse, or is bleeding severely.

Fortunately, most of the victims you encounter will be conscious. Very likely, they will be able to indicate what is wrong by speaking to you or by gesturing. You will be able to ask them questions. But when a person cannot be aroused, it is difficult to know what is wrong, besides the fact that he or she is unconscious. Unconsciousness is a signal that the victim's life is threatened. You need to have someone call for an ambulance while you continue to check the victim to see if he or she is breathing, has a pulse, or is bleeding severely.

You may have to care for a person who is unconscious but who is breathing normally and has a pulse. For example, a person might have hit his or her head in a fall or just fainted. In such cases, make sure someone has called the local emergency number. There is no need to move the person as long as he or she is breathing adequately. If the person vomits, roll him or her onto one side and clear the mouth and throat. If the person stops breathing, position the person on his or her back and breathe for the person as described later in this article. If you are alone and have to leave the person for any reason, such as to call for help, position the person on the side in case he or she vomits while you are gone.

Most often, unconsciousness is a signal that a victim may have other life-threatening conditions. A person who is unconscious will soon die if breathing stops and if the heart stops. You must discover

0 minutes: Breathing stops. Heart will soon stop beating.

4 - 6 minutes: Brain damage possible.

6 - 10 minutes: Brain damage likely.

Over 10 minutes: Irreversible brain damage certain.

Time is critical in life-threatening emergencies. Unless the brain gets oxygen within minutes of when breathing stops, brain damage or death will occur.

and care for these conditions as quickly as possible.

Breathing Emergencies

The body requires a constant supply of oxygen to survive. When you breathe air in through the nose and mouth, it travels down the throat, through the windpipe, and into the lungs. This pathway from the nose and mouth to the lungs is commonly called the airway. Once air reaches the lungs, oxygen in the air is transferred to the blood. The blood transports the oxygen to the brain, and heart, as well as to all other parts of the body.

Certain emergencies are life-threatening because they greatly

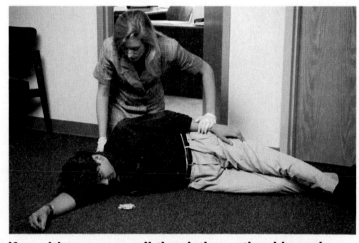

If vomiting occurs, roll the victim on the side, and clear the mouth of any matter.

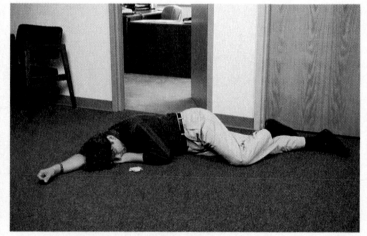

If you are alone and must leave an unconscious victim, position the person on one side in case he or she vomits while you are gone.

OXYGEN IS VITAL TO LIFE

The body requires a constant supply of oxygen to survive. When you breathe air in through the nose and mouth, it travels down the throat, through the windpipe, and into the lungs. This path from the nose and mouth to the lungs is called the airway.

When the air you breathe reaches the lungs, oxygen from the air is transferred to the blood and is circulated to all parts of the body through large blood vessels called arteries.

Injuries and illnesses that affect breathing or the action of the heart or cause bleeding can interrupt the supply of oxygen. When enough oxygen does not reach the lungs or does not circulate properly in the body, it is a life-threatening emergency. You must act immediately.

SIGNALS

OF

BREATHING EMERGENCIES

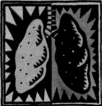

Breathing is unusually slow or rapid.

Breaths are unusually deep or shallow.

Victim is gasping for breath.

Victim is wheezing, gurgling, or making high-pitched noises.

Victim's skin is unusually moist.

Victim's skin has a flushed, pale, or bluish appearance.

Victim feels short of breath.

Victim feels dizzy or light-headed.

Victim feels pain in chest or tingling in hands or feet.

reduce or eliminate the body's supply of oxygen. For instance, when a person has difficulty breathing, that person's body may not get enough oxygen. When breathing stops or when the heart stops, the body gets none. Unless the brain gets oxygen within minutes of when breathing stops, brain damage or death will occur.

A breathing problem so severe that it threatens the victim's life is a breathing emergency. In "Checking the Victim," you learned that you have to check to find out whether an unconscious victim is breathing. You also learned that if the victim is breathing, you must determine if he or she is having difficulty breathing.

Breathing emergencies can be caused by injury or illness. For example, if the heart stops beating, breathing will stop. Choking and injury or disease in areas of the brain that control breathing can disturb or stop breathing. In an unconscious person, a likely reason for breathing to stop is that the tongue falls back in the throat and blocks the airway.

Damage to the muscles or bones of the chest can make breathing painful or difficult. Electric shock and drowning can cause breathing to stop. Severe reactions to certain poisons, drugs, insect stings, and foods can also cause breathing emergencies. Other causes include anxiety, excitement, and conditions such as asthma.

Asthma, for example, is a condition that narrows the air passages. This makes breathing difficult, which is frightening. Asthma may be triggered by a reaction to food, pollen, medications, or insect stings. Emotional distress or physical activity can also bring on an asthma attack. People with asthma can usually control an attack with medication. They may carry this medication with them.

Asthma is more common in children and young adults than in older people. You can often tell when a person is having an asthma attack by the wheezing noises he or she makes when breathing.

Hyperventilation occurs when a person breathes faster than normal. It is often the result of fear or anxiety and is most likely to occur in people who are tense and nervous. However, it can also be caused by head injuries, severe bleeding, or illnesses, such as high fever, heart failure, lung disease, and diabetic emergencies. Asthma and exercise also can trigger hyperventilation.

People who are hyperventilating have rapid, shallow breathing. They feel as if they can't get enough air. Often they are afraid and anxious or seem confused. They may say that they feel dizzy or their fingers and toes feel numb and tingly.

Allergic reactions can also cause breathing problems. At first, the reaction may appear only as a rash and a feeling of tightness in the chest and throat, but this condition can become life-threatening. The victim's face, neck, and tongue may swell, closing the airway.

Severe allergic reactions can be caused by insect stings, certain foods, and medications. People who know they have severe allergic reactions to certain things may have learned to avoid them. They may also carry medication to reverse the reaction. If not cared for at once, a severe allergic reaction can become life-threatening.

Even though there are many causes of breathing emergencies, you do not need to know the exact cause of a breathing emergency to care for it. You do need to be able to recognize when a person is having trouble breathing or is not breathing at all.

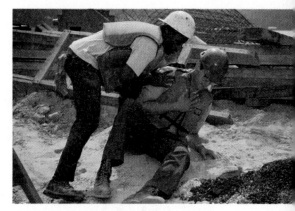

A person who is having trouble breathing may breathe more easily in a sitting position.

If a Person Has Trouble Breathing

Normal breathing is easy and quiet. The person doesn't look as if he or she is working hard or struggling to breathe. The person isn't making noise when breathing. Breaths aren't fast or far apart. Breathing doesn't cause the person pain.

The kind of breathing emergency you are most likely to encounter is a conscious person who is having trouble breathing. You can usually identify a breathing problem by watching and listening to the person's breathing and by asking the person how he or she feels. You should also check the victim's skin appearance.

People with breathing problems may look as if they can't catch

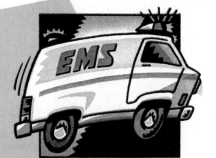

When breathing is too fast, slow, noisy, or painful,

CALL FOR AN AMBULANCE
IMMEDIATELY!

their breath. They may gasp for air. They may appear to breathe faster or slower than normal. Their breaths may be unusually deep or shallow. They may make unusual noises, such as wheezing or gurgling. They may make high-pitched noises in their throats. They may have difficulty talking to you or may not be able to talk at all. Their skin, at first, may be damp and look flushed. Later, it may look pale or bluish because their blood is getting low on oxygen.

People with breathing problems may say they feel dizzy or light-headed. They may feel pain in the chest or tingling in the hands and feet. They may be afraid or anxious.

Recognizing the signals of breathing problems and giving care are often the keys to preventing these problems from becoming more serious emergencies. A breathing problem such as choking can cause the victim to stop breathing entirely. Difficulty breathing can be the first signal of a more serious emergency, such as a heart problem.

If a person is having trouble breathing, help him or her rest in a comfortable position. Usually, sitting is more comfortable than lying down because breathing is easier in that position. If the victim is conscious, check for other conditions. Remember that a person having breathing problems may find it hard to talk. Ask bystanders if they know about the victim's condition. The victim can nod to answer yes-or-no questions. Try to reassure the victim and reduce anxiety. This may make his or her breathing easier.

If the victim is breathing rapidly (hyperventilating) and you are sure it is caused by emotion, such as ex-

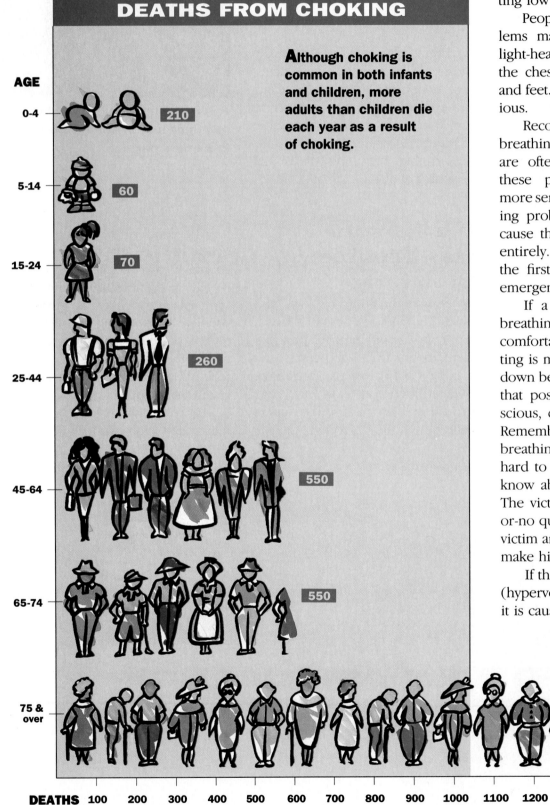

DEATHS FROM CHOKING

Although choking is common in both infants and children, more adults than children die each year as a result of choking.

AGE

0-4 — 210

5-14 — 60

15-24 — 70

25-44 — 260

45-64 — 550

65-74 — 550

75 & over — 1,500

DEATHS 100 200 300 400 500 600 700 800 900 1000 1100 1200 1300 1400 1500 1600

National Safety Council. *Accident Facts,* 1991 Edition.

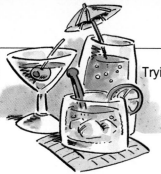

Trying to swallow large pieces of poorly chewed food

Drinking alcohol before or during meals (Alcohol dulls the nerves that aid swallowing.)

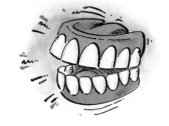

Common Causes of Choking

Wearing dentures (Dentures make it difficult to sense whether food is fully chewed before it is swallowed.)

Eating while talking excitedly or laughing, or eating too fast

Walking, playing, or running with food or objects in mouth

citement or fear, tell the victim to relax and breathe slowly. A victim who is hyperventilating from emotion may resume normal breathing if he or she is reassured and calmed down. If the victim's breathing still doesn't slow down, the victim could have a serious problem.

When breathing is too fast, slow, noisy, or painful, call for an ambulance immediately.

If a Person Is Choking

Choking is a common breathing emergency. A conscious person who is choking has the airway blocked by a piece of food or another object. The airway may be partially or completely blocked. A person whose airway is completely blocked can't breathe at all. With a partially blocked airway, the victim is often still able to breathe, although breathing is difficult.

A person with a partially blocked airway can get enough air in and out of the lungs to cough or to make wheezing sounds. The person may also get enough air to speak.

If the choking person is coughing forcefully, let him or her try to cough up the object. A person who

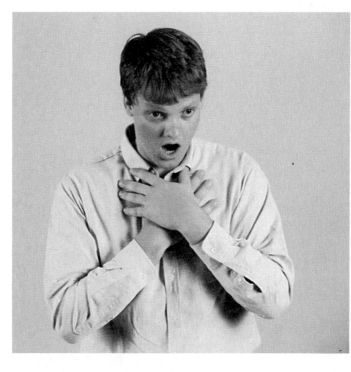

Clutching the throat with one or both hands is universally recognized as a distress signal for choking.

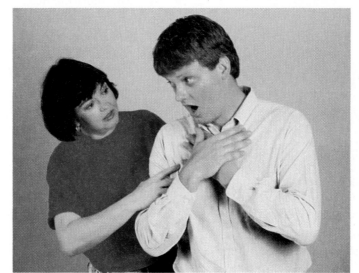

If a choking person is coughing forcefully, encourage him or her to continue coughing.

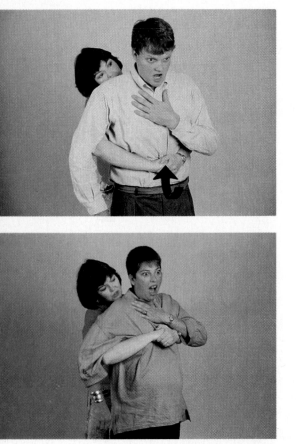

A person who cannot speak, cough forcefully, or breathe is choking. Give quick upward thrusts to the abdomen, just above the navel, until the airway is cleared (*top*). Give chest thrusts when a choking victim is too big for you to reach around or if the victim is noticeably pregnant.

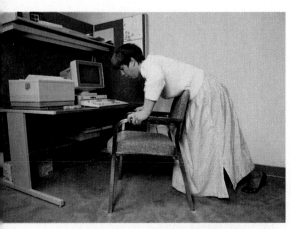

To give yourself abdominal thrusts, press your abdomen onto a firm object, such as the back of a chair.

is getting enough air to cough or speak is getting enough air to breathe. Stay with the person and encourage him or her to continue coughing. However, if the person continues to cough without coughing up the object, call for an ambulance.

A partially blocked airway can very quickly become completely blocked. A person whose airway is completely blocked can't speak, cough forcefully, or breathe. Sometimes the person may cough weakly or make high-pitched noises. This tells you the person isn't getting enough air to stay alive. Act at once! Have a bystander call for an ambulance while you begin to give care.

When someone is choking, you must get the airway open quickly. To do this, give a series of quick, hard thrusts to the victim's abdomen. These abdominal thrusts are also called the Heimlich maneuver. These upward thrusts push the abdomen in, putting pressure on the lungs and airway. This forces the air in the lungs to push the object out of the airway—like the cork from a bottle of champagne.

To give abdominal thrusts, stand behind the victim. Wrap your arms around the victim's waist. Make a fist with one hand and place the thumb side against the middle of the victim's abdomen just above the navel but below the rib cage. Grab your fist with your other hand and give quick, inward and upward thrusts into the abdomen. Repeat these thrusts until the object is forced out or the victim becomes unconscious. If the victim becomes unconscious, follow the procedures for checking an unconscious victim.

If a conscious victim is too big for you to reach around and give effective abdominal thrusts, give chest thrusts. Give chest thrusts to an obviously pregnant victim.

Chest thrusts for a conscious

SKILL SHEET

Give Abdominal Thrusts

If, when you check, the person is unable to speak, cough, or breathe. . .

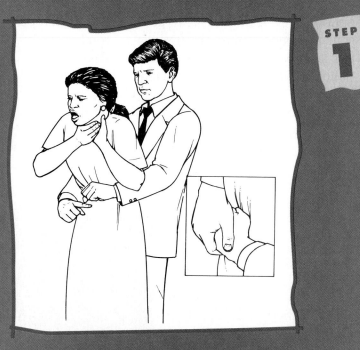

STEP 1

Place thumb side of fist against middle of abdomen just above the navel. Grasp fist with other hand.

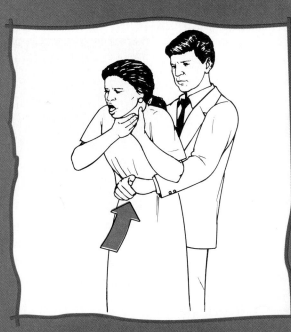

STEP 2

Give quick, upward thrusts.

Repeat until object is coughed up or person becomes unconscious.

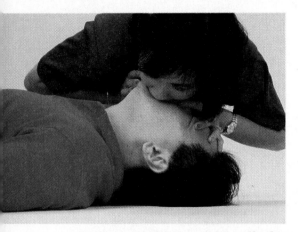

To give rescue breathing, tilt the head back, lift the chin, and pinch the nose shut. Breathe into the victim's mouth.

victim are like abdominal thrusts, except for the placement of your hands. Place your fist against the center of the victim's breastbone. Grab it with your other hand and give quick thrusts into the chest.

If you are alone and choking, you can give yourself abdominal thrusts with your hands. Another option is to lean over and press your abdomen against any firm object such as the back of a chair, a railing, or the kitchen sink. Don't lean over anything with a sharp edge or corner that might hurt you.

If a Person Is Not Breathing

If a person's breathing stops or is restricted long enough, that person will become unconscious, the heart will stop beating, and blood will no longer circulate in the body. Other body systems will quickly fail.

When a person stops breathing, you have to breathe for that person. This is called rescue breathing. It is a way of breathing air into a person that supplies him or her with the oxygen needed to stay alive. Rescue breathing is given to anyone who is unconscious and not breathing but has a pulse.

When a person stops breathing, you have to breathe for that person. This is called

RESCUE BREATHING

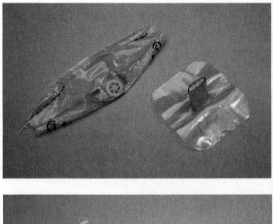

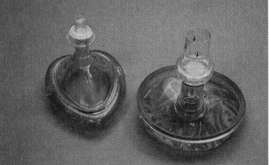

A face shield (*top*) or mask (*bottom*), when placed between your mouth and nose and the victim's, can help prevent you from contacting a person's saliva or other body fluids.

WHEN YOU GIVE RESCUE BREATHING,

breathe *slowly* into the victim,
only until the chest
gently rises.

To give rescue breathing, begin by tilting the head back and lifting the chin to move the tongue away from the back of the throat. This opens the airway, the path that air travels from the nose and mouth to the lungs. Place your ear next to the victim's mouth. Check for breathing by looking at the chest and listening and feeling for breathing for about 5 seconds. If you can't see, hear, or feel any signs of breathing, you must begin to breathe for the victim.

Pinch the victim's nose shut and make a tight seal around the victim's mouth with your mouth. Breathe slowly and gently into the victim until you see the chest rise. Give two breaths, each lasting about 1½ seconds. Pause between breaths to let the air flow out. Watch the victim's chest rise each time you give a breath to make sure your breaths are going in.

Check for a pulse after giving these 2 initial slow breaths. If you feel a pulse but the victim is still not breathing, give one breath about every 5 seconds. You can time the breaths by counting, "one one-thousand, two one-thousand, three one-thousand." Then take a breath on "four one-thousand" and breathe into the victim on "five one-thousand." Counting this way ensures that you give one breath about every 5 seconds. After 10 to 12 breaths, recheck the pulse to make sure the heart is still beating. If the victim has a pulse but is still not breathing, continue rescue breathing. Recheck the pulse about every 10 to 12 breaths. Continue rescue breathing until one of the following happens:

- The victim begins to breathe without your help.
- The victim has no pulse (begin CPR).
- Another trained rescuer takes over for you.
- You are too tired to go on.

You might not feel comfortable with the thought of giving rescue breathing, especially to someone you don't know. Disease transmission is an understandable worry, even though the chances of getting a disease from giving rescue breathing are extremely low. Barriers, such as shields and masks you put between your mouth and nose and the victim's, can help protect you from blood and other body fluids, such as saliva. The devices with one-way valves help protect you from breathing the air the

SKILL SHEET

If Person is Not Breathing...

Give Rescue Breathing

The emergency number has been called. If, when you check, the person is not breathing. . .

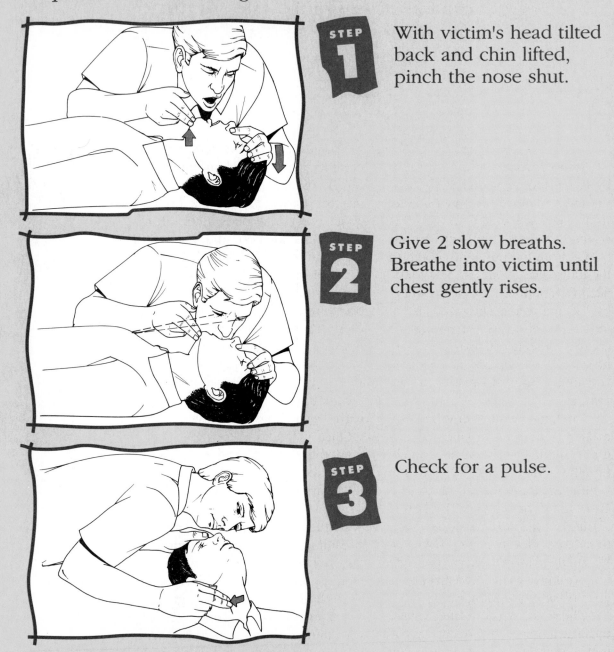

STEP 1 With victim's head tilted back and chin lifted, pinch the nose shut.

STEP 2 Give 2 slow breaths. Breathe into victim until chest gently rises.

STEP 3 Check for a pulse.

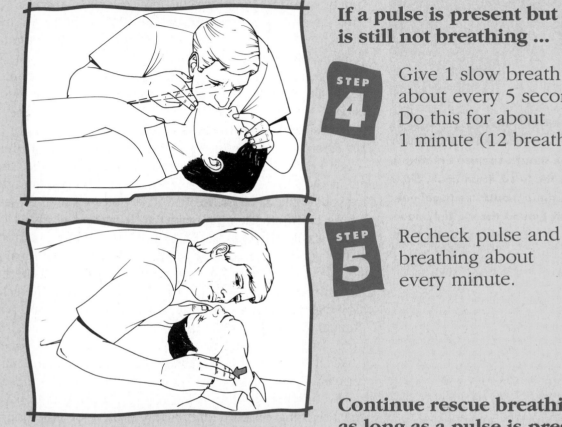

If a pulse is present but person is still not breathing ...

STEP 4
Give 1 slow breath about every 5 seconds. Do this for about 1 minute (12 breaths).

STEP 5
Recheck pulse and breathing about every minute.

Continue rescue breathing as long as a pulse is present but person is not breathing.

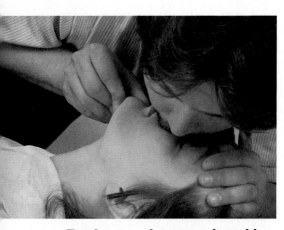

To give mouth-to-nose breathing, keep the head tilted back, close the victim's mouth, and seal your mouth around the victim's nose. Breathe into the nose.

victim exhales. Some devices are small enough to fit in your pocket or in the glove compartment of your car. You can also keep one in your first aid kit.

When you are giving rescue breathing, you want to avoid getting air in the victim's stomach instead of the lungs. This may happen if you breathe too long, breathe too hard, or don't open the airway far enough.

To avoid getting air into the victim's stomach, keep the victim's head tilted back. Breathe *slowly* into the victim, just enough to make the chest rise. Each breath should last about 1½ seconds. Pause between breaths long enough for the air in the victim to come out and for you to take another breath.

Air in the stomach can make the victim vomit. When an unconscious victim vomits, the contents of the stomach can get into the lungs and block breathing. Air in the stomach also makes it harder for the diaphragm, the large muscle that controls breathing, to move. This makes it harder for the lungs to fill with air.

Even when you are giving rescue breathing properly, the victim may vomit. If this happens, turn the victim onto one side and wipe the

mouth clean. If possible, use a protective barrier, such as latex gloves, gauze, or even a handkerchief, when cleaning out the mouth. Then roll the victim on his or her back again and continue with rescue breathing.

Sometimes you may not be able to make a tight enough seal over a victim's mouth. For example, the person's jaw or mouth may be injured or shut too tightly to open or your mouth may be too small to cover the victim's mouth. If you can't make a tight seal, you can breathe into the nose. With the head tilted back, close the mouth by pushing on the chin. Seal your mouth around the victim's nose and breathe into the nose. If possible, open the victim's mouth between breaths to let the air out.

On rare occasions, you may see an opening in a victim's neck as you tilt the head back to check for breathing. This victim may have had an operation to remove part of the windpipe. The victim breathes through this opening, which is called a stoma, instead of through the mouth or nose. This victim will probably also have some medical alert identification, such as a bracelet, identifying this condition. Look, listen, and feel for breathing with

You may need to perform rescue breathing on a victim with a stoma, an opening in the front of the neck *(left)*. To check for breathing, look, listen, and feel for breaths with your ear over the stoma *(middle)*. To give rescue breathing, seal your mouth around the stoma and breathe into the victim *(right)*.

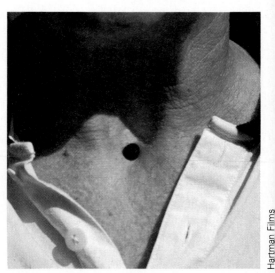

Hartman Films

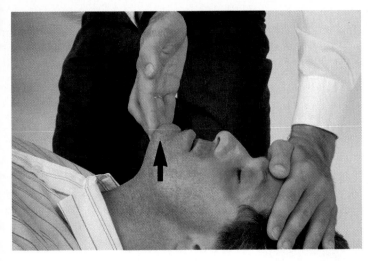

your ear over the stoma. To give rescue breathing to this victim, breathe into the stoma at the same rate as you would breathe into the mouth.

You may have to care for an unconscious person who has nearly drowned. If so, get the person out of the water as quickly as possible. If the victim is not breathing, you will have to breathe for him or her.

Finally, be especially careful when a victim may have a head, neck, or back injury. These can result, for example, from a fall from a height, an automobile collision, or a diving mishap. If you suspect such an injury, try not to move the victim's head and neck. Try to lift the chin without tilting the head when checking breathing and giving rescue breathing. If you are trying to breathe for that person and your breaths don't go in, tilt the head back only slightly. This is all that is usually needed to let air go in. If air still doesn't go in, tilt the head a little more. It is unlikely that tilting the head slightly will further damage the neck. Remember that the nonbreathing victim's greatest need is for air.

If Air Does Not Go In

If you do not see the victim's chest rise and fall as you give

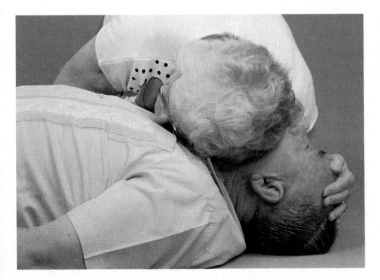

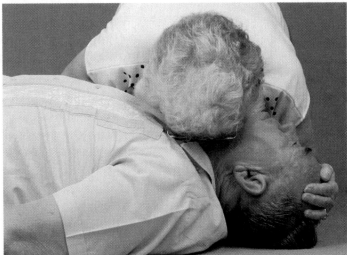

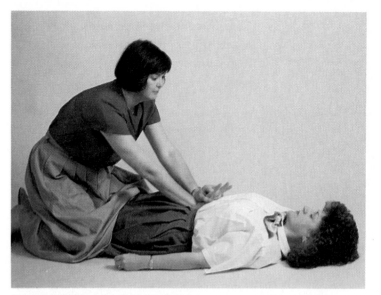

To give abdominal thrusts to an unconscious victim, place the heel of your hands just above the navel with your fingers pointing toward the victim's head and give quick, upward thrusts.

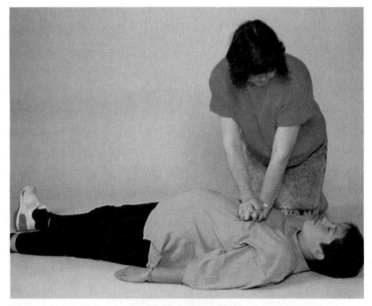

If an unconscious victim is pregnant, give chest thrusts. Kneel to one side of the victim, place the heel of one hand in the center of the breastbone and give quick, downward thrusts.

breaths, you might not have tilted the head far enough back. Retilt the victim's head and repeat the breaths. If your breaths still don't go in, the airway is probably blocked. The airway can become blocked by the tongue falling back in the throat, by food, by an object such as a coin, or by fluids such as blood or saliva.

If you have tried to give 2 slow breaths, retilted the head, and tried again with no success, you must try to clear the airway. This is done by giving up to 5 abdominal thrusts and trying to sweep the object out with your finger.

To give abdominal thrusts to an unconscious victim, straddle one or both of the victim's legs. Place the heel of one hand on the middle of the abdomen just above the navel. Place the other hand on top of the first. Point the fingers of both hands directly toward the victim's head. Give quick thrusts toward the head and into the abdomen.

After giving 5 thrusts, lift the victim's lower jaw and tongue with your fingers and thumb. Slide one finger down the inside of the victim's cheek and try to hook the object out. Be careful not to push it further down. Then reattempt your 2 slow breaths. If you still can't get air into the victim, repeat thrusts, finger sweeps, and breaths. Continue this sequence until the object is removed and you can breathe into the victim.

To give chest thrusts to an unconscious victim whose airway is blocked, kneel to the side of the victim. Place the heel of one hand on the center of the victim's breastbone. Place the other hand on top of it. Give up to 5 quick thrusts. Each thrust should push the chest down about 1½ inches. Then let the chest come up.

Once you are able to get air into the victim, continue to check the victim by feeling for a pulse. If the victim is not breathing, give rescue breathing. If the victim does not have a pulse, give CPR.

Stop giving abdominal or chest thrusts at once if the object comes out or the victim begins to breathe or cough. Make sure the object is out of the airway and watch to see that the person is breathing freely again. Even after the object is coughed up, the person may have breathing problems that you don't notice right away. Also, abdominal thrusts and chest thrusts can cause internal injuries. Therefore, whenever thrusts are used to dislodge an object, the victim should be taken to the nearest hospital emergency department for follow-up care, even if he or she seems to be breathing without difficulty.

SKILL SHEET

If Air Does Not Go In...

IF AN UNCONSCIOUS PERSON'S AIRWAY IS BLOCKED,

it is more important to get air in than to get the object out.

Give Abdominal Thrusts

The emergency number has been called. If, when you check, the person is not breathing and your breaths do not go in . . .

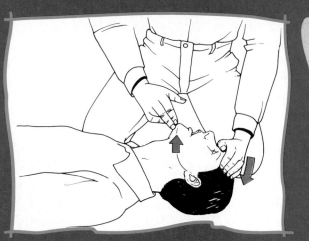

STEP 1

Retilt person's head.

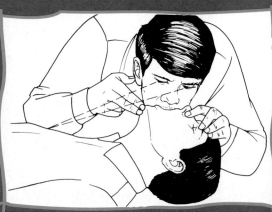

STEP 2

Give breaths again.

If air still won't go in ...

STEP 3

Place heel of one hand against middle of abdomen just above the navel.

STEP 4 Give up to 5 abdominal thrusts.

STEP 5 Lift jaw and tongue and sweep out mouth.

STEP 6 Tilt head back, lift chin, and give breaths again.

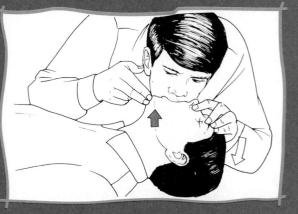

Repeat breaths, thrusts, and sweeps until breaths go in.

It is estimated that 70 million Americans suffer some form of cardiovascular disease. Nearly 1 million deaths each year are attributed to cardiovascular disease. Of these, more than half result from heart attacks. The good news is that deaths caused by heart attacks have dropped by over 30 percent and deaths caused by stroke have dropped 50 percent over the past 20 years. An increased awareness of what it means to lead a healthier life has prompted many Americans to make heart-healthy changes in their lives. It is estimated that these changes, including stopping smoking, eating right, and getting regular exercise, have saved as many as 250,000 lives each year.

the HEART of the matter

The heart is a fascinating organ. It beats more than 3 billion times in an average lifetime. The heart is about the size of a fist and lies between the lungs in the middle of the chest. It pumps blood throughout the body. The ribs, breastbone, and the spine protect it from injury. The heart is separated into right and left halves. Blood that contains little or no oxygen enters the right side of the heart and is pumped to the lungs. The blood picks up oxygen in the

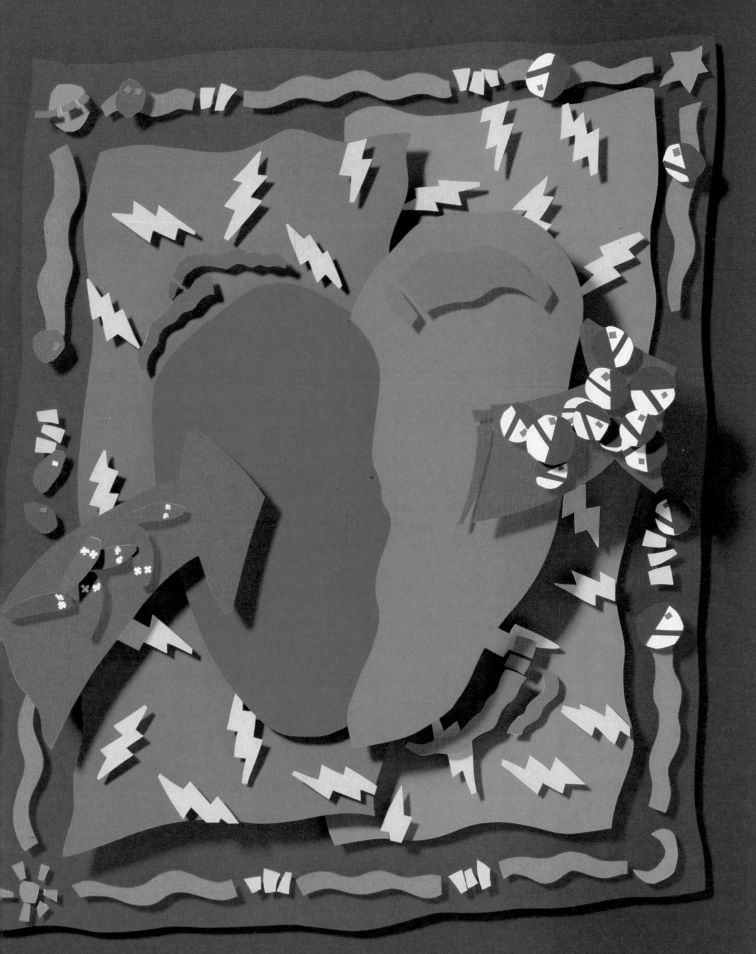

lungs when you breathe. The oxygen-rich blood then goes to the left side of the heart and is pumped to all parts of the body.

The heart needs a constant supply of oxygen. Blood vessels called arteries supply the heart with oxygen-rich blood. If the heart does not get this blood, it will not work properly. When the heart is behaving normally, it beats evenly and easily, with a steady rhythm. When damage to the heart causes it to stop working effectively, a person experiences a heart attack. A heart attack can cause the heart to beat in an irregular way. This may prevent blood from circulating effectively. When the heart doesn't work properly, normal breathing can be disrupted or stopped. A heart attack can also cause the heart to stop beating entirely. This condition is called cardiac arrest.

Any chest pain that is severe, lasts longer than 10 minutes, or persists even during rest requires immediate medical care.

Signals of Heart Problems

A heart attack has some common signals. You should be able to recognize these signals so that you can provide proper care.

The major signal is pain or discomfort in the chest that does not go away. Unfortunately, it isn't always easy to tell heart attack pain from the pain of indigestion, muscle spasms, or other conditions. This often causes people to delay obtaining medical care. Brief, stabbing pain or pain that gets worse when you bend or breathe deeply is not usually caused by a heart problem.

The pain associated with a heart attack can range from discomfort to an unbearable crushing sensation in the chest. The victim may describe it as pressure, squeezing, tightness, aching, or heaviness in the chest. Often the victim feels pain in the center of the chest. It may spread to the shoulder, arm, neck, jaw, or back. The pain is constant. It is usually not relieved by resting, changing position, or taking medicine. Any chest pain that is severe, lasts longer than 10 minutes, or persists even during rest requires medical care at once.

Another signal of a heart attack is difficulty breathing. The victim may be breathing faster than normal because the body tries to get much-needed oxygen to the heart. The victim's skin may be pale or bluish, especially around the face. The face may also be damp with sweat. Some heart attack victims

The right side receives oxygen-poor blood (blue) from the body and sends it to the lungs where it picks up oxygen. The left side receives oxygen-rich blood (red) from the lungs and pumps it out through the body. One-way valves direct the flow of blood through the heart.

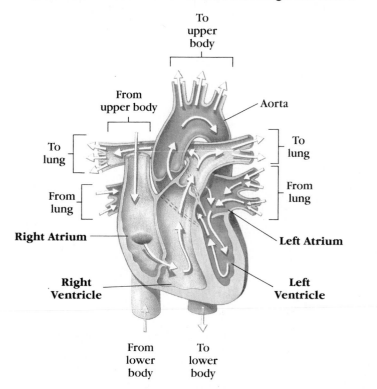

To upper body

From upper body

Aorta

To lung

To lung

From lung

From lung

Right Atrium

Left Atrium

Right Ventricle

Left Ventricle

From lower body

To lower body

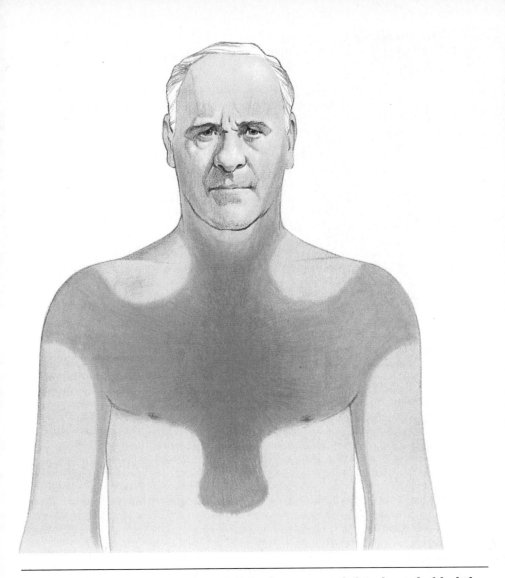

Heart attack pain is most often felt in the center of the chest, behind the breastbone. It may spread to the shoulder, arm, or jaw.

sweat heavily. These signals are caused by the stress put on the body when the heart does not work as it should.

Some people with heart disease may have chest pain or pressure that comes and goes. This type of pain is called angina pectoris, a medical term for pain in the chest. It develops when the heart needs more oxygen than it gets because the arteries leading to the heart are too narrow. When a person with angina is exercising, excited, or emotionally upset, the heart might not get enough oxygen. This lack of oxygen can cause chest pain.

Unlike the pain of a heart attack, the pain associated with angina rarely lasts more than 10 minutes. A person who knows he or she has angina may tell you so. Individuals with angina usually have medicine to take to stop the pain. Stopping physical activity or easing the distress and taking the medicine usually stops the pain of angina.

It is important to recognize the signals of a heart attack and act on them. Any heart attack may lead to cardiac arrest! Prompt action may prevent it. A heart attack victim whose heart is still beating has a far

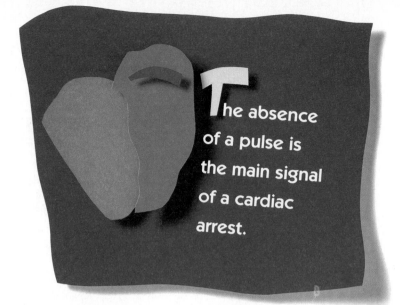

The absence of a pulse is the main signal of a cardiac arrest.

better chance of living than one whose heart has stopped. Most people who die of heart attack die within 2 hours after the first signals appear. Many could have been saved if people on the scene or the victim had been aware of the signals and acted promptly. Early treatment with certain medications, for example, can help minimize damage to the heart after a heart attack.

Many heart attack victims delay getting care. Nearly half of them wait for 2 hours or more before going to the hospital. Often they do not realize they are having a heart attack. They may say the signals are just muscle soreness or indigestion.

Remember, the key signal of a heart attack is chest pain that does not go away. If the pain is severe or does not go away in 10 minutes, call for an ambulance at once. A heart attack victim will probably deny that any signal is serious. Do not let this influence you. If you think the victim might be having a heart attack, you must act quickly. Call your emergency number!

Care for a Heart Attack

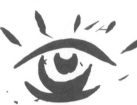

Recognize the signals of a heart attack.

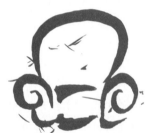

Convince the victim to stop activity and rest.

Help the victim to rest comfortably.

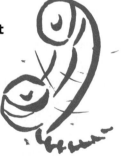

Try to obtain information about the victim's condition.

Comfort the victim.

Call the local emergency number for help.

Assist with medication, if prescribed.

Monitor the victim's condition.

Be prepared to give CPR if the victim's heart stops beating.

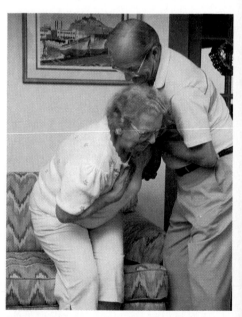

Have a victim with severe chest pain stop and rest. Many victims find it easier to breathe while sitting.

In Case of a Heart Attack

Whenever you suspect that a person is having a heart attack, have the victim stop whatever he or she is doing and rest. Many heart attack victims find it easier to breathe while sitting. Talk to bystanders and the victim, if possible, to learn more. If the victim is having persistent chest pain, ask the victim when the pain started. Ask what brought the pain on, if anything lessens it, what it feels like, and where it hurts.

Ask the victim if he or she has a history of heart disease. Some people with heart disease have medicine to take for it. You can help by getting the medicine for the victim. If you still think the victim may be having a heart attack or if you aren't sure, call for an ambulance. Have a bystander call, or make the call yourself if you're alone. To survive a heart attack, a person needs advanced medical care just as soon as possible! Call your local emergency number before the victim gets worse and the heart stops.

Be calm and reassuring when caring for a heart attack victim. When you comfort the victim, it helps make him or her less anxious and more comfortable. Watch carefully for any changes in the way the victim looks and behaves. Since the victim may go into cardiac arrest, be prepared to give cardiopulmonary resuscitation (CPR).

When the Heart Stops Beating

When the heart stops beating or beats too poorly to circulate blood properly, it is called cardiac arrest. When cardiac arrest happens, breathing soon stops. Cardiac arrest is life-threatening. Every year, more than 300,000 victims die of cardiac arrest before they reach a hospital.

Heart disease is the most common cause of cardiac arrest. Other causes include drowning, choking, and certain drugs. These causes, as well as severe injury, brain damage, and severe electric shock, can cause the heart to stop. Cardiac arrest can happen suddenly, without the signals usually seen in a heart attack.

A person in cardiac arrest is unconscious, is not breathing, and has no pulse. The absence of a pulse is the main signal of cardiac arrest. No matter how hard you try, you won't be able to find a pulse. No pulse means no blood is going to the brain. Since blood carries oxygen, no oxygen is going to the brain and the brain will die.

Even though a victim is not breathing and has no pulse, the cells of the brain and of other important organs continue to live for a short time—until the oxygen in the blood is used up. Such a victim needs CPR at once. CPR is a combination of chest compressions and

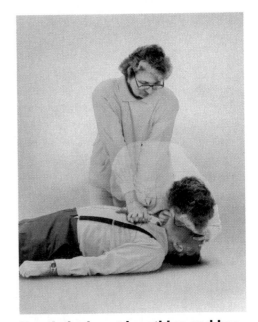

If a victim is not breathing and has no pulse, he or she needs CPR. CPR is a combination of chest compressions and rescue breathing.

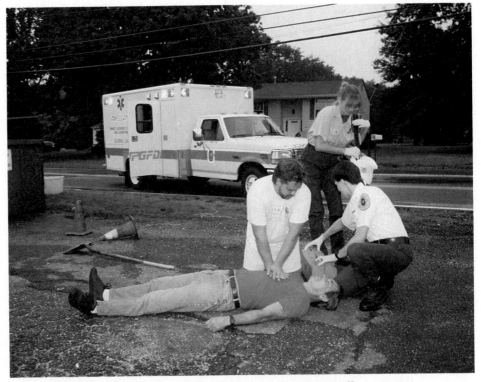

CPR alone is not enough to help someone survive cardiac arrest. Advanced medical care is needed as soon as possible.

rescue breathing. As you read earlier, rescue breathing supplies oxygen. The presence of a pulse means that the heart is circulating this oxygen to the body through the blood. When the heart isn't beating, chest compressions are needed to circulate the oxygen. Given together, rescue breathing and chest compressions take over for the heart and lungs. CPR increases a cardiac arrest victim's chances of survival by keeping the brain supplied with oxygen until the victim can get medical care. Without CPR, the brain begins to die in as little as 4 minutes.

However, CPR provides only about one third the normal blood flow to the brain. CPR alone is not enough to help someone survive cardiac arrest. Advanced medical care is needed as soon as possible. This is why it is so important to call for an ambulance immediately! Trained emergency personnel can provide special care for cardiac arrest. They can use a device called a defibrillator, which sends an electric shock through the chest. The shock enables the heart to begin beating properly again. They can also give medication.

A Matter of Choice

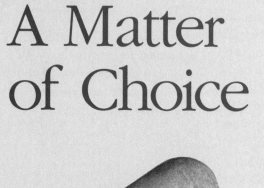

Your 75-year-old grandfather is living with your family. He has a terminal illness and is frequently in the hospital. He has no hope of regaining his health.

One afternoon, you go to his room to give him lunch. As you start to talk to him, you realize he has stopped breathing. You check for a pulse. He has none. You are suddenly faced with the fact that your grandfather is no longer alive . . . he's dead. You ask yourself . . . What do I do?

No one can tell you what to do. No one can advise you. No one can predict the outcome. The decision to try to help your grandfather by giving CPR is a personal one that you must make.

Your mind tells you to give CPR, yet your heart tells you not to. Various questions race through your mind. Can I face the fact I am losing someone I love? Shouldn't I always try to give CPR? What would his life be like after resuscitation? What would grandfather want?

It is important to realize that it is OK to withhold CPR when a terminally ill person is dying. Nature takes its course, and, in some cases, people feel they have lived full lives and are prepared for death. Talking to your grandfather about preferences *before* a crisis occurs can help you with such decisions.

How would this situation have changed if your family and grandfather had planned for this possibility? For instance, what would have happened if your grandfather had given instructions in advance?

Instructions that describe a person's wishes about medical treatment are called advance directives. These instructions are used when the person can no longer make his or her own health-care decisions. If your grandfather is able to make decisions, advance directives do not interfere with his right to do so.

As provided by the federal Patient Self-Determination Act, adults who are admitted to a hospital or a health-care facility or who receive assistance from certain organizations that receive funds from Medicare and

A person in cardiac arrest needs defibrillation as soon as possible. A person has the best chance of surviving cardiac arrest if a bystander gives CPR at once and EMS personnel follow up rapidly with defibrillation.

It is very important to start CPR promptly and continue it until EMS personnel arrive. Any delay in calling for an ambulance and starting CPR makes it less likely the victim will survive. Remember, you are the first link in the victim's chain of survival.

No one is exactly sure how chest compressions work. It is generally thought that chest compressions create pressure in the chest that causes blood to circulate through the body. For compressions to be most effective, the vic-

Medicaid have the right to make fundamental choices about their own care. They must be told about their right to make decisions about the level of life support that would be provided in an emergency situation. They would be offered the opportunity to make these choices at the time of admission.

Verbal conversations with relatives, friends, or physicians, while the patient is still capable of making decisions, are the most common form of advance directives. However, because conversations may not be recalled accurately, the courts consider written directives more trustworthy.

Two examples of written advance directives are living wills and durable powers of attorney for health care. The types of health-care decisions covered by these documents vary depending on where you live. Talking with a legal professional can help determine which advance directive options are available in your state and what they do and do not cover.

If your grandfather had established a living will, directions for health care would be in place before he became unable to communicate his wishes. The instructions that can be included in this document vary from state to state. A living will generally allows a person to refuse only medical care that "merely prolongs the process of dying," such as with a terminal illness.

If your grandfather had established a durable power of attorney for health care, the document would authorize someone to make medical decisions for him in any situation in which he could no longer make them for himself. This authorized person is called a *health care surrogate* or *proxy*. This surrogate, with the information given by the patient's physician, may consent to or refuse medical treatment on the patient's behalf. In this case, he or she would support the needs and wishes that affect the health-care decisions and the advance directives of your grandfather.

A doctor could formalize your grandfather's preferences by writing "Do Not Resuscitate" (DNR) orders in your grandfather's medical records. Such orders would state that if your grandfather's heartbeat or breathing stops, he should not be resuscitated. The choice in deciding on DNR orders may be covered in a living will or in the durable power of attorney for health care.

Appointing someone to act as a health care surrogate along with writing down your instructions is the best way to formalize your wishes about medical care.

Some of these documents can be obtained through a personal physician, attorney, or various state and health-care organizations. A lawyer is not always needed to execute advance directives. However, if you have any questions concerning advance directives, it is wise to obtain legal advice.

Copies of advance directives should be provided to all personal physicians, family members, and the person chosen as the health care surrogate. Tell them what documents have been prepared and where the original and other copies are located. Discuss the docu-ment with all parties so they understand the intent of all requests. Keep these documents updated.

Keep in mind that advance directives are not limited to elderly people or people with terminal illnesses. Advance directives should be considered by anyone who has decided the care he or she would like to have provided. An unexpected illness or injury could create a need for decisions at any time.

Knowing about living wills, durable powers of attorneys for health care, and DNR orders can help you prepare for difficult decisions. If you are interested in learning more about your rights and the options available to you in your state, contact a legal professional.

REFERENCES
1. Hospital Shared Services of Colorado, Stockard Inventory Program. *Your Right to Make Health Care Decisions.* Denver, Colorado, 1991.
2. Title 42 United States Code, Section 1395 cc (a)(1)(Q)(A) Patient Self-Determination Act.

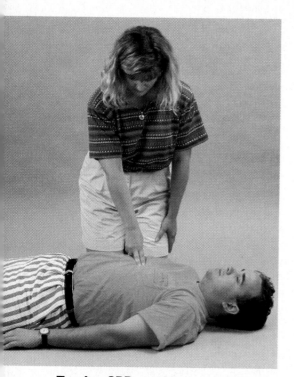

To give CPR, position yourself so that you can give rescue breaths and chest compressions without having to move.

tim should be lying flat, on his or her back, and on a level surface. If a person is in bed, move the person to the floor. CPR doesn't work as well if the victim is sitting up or is on a soft surface like a mattress.

After determining that a victim does not have a pulse, begin chest compressions and rescue breathing. To give chest compressions, kneel beside the victim. Place yourself midway between the head and the chest in order to move easily from giving compressions to giving breaths. Lean over the chest and position your hands. The correct hand and body position lets you give the most effective compressions without tiring you too quickly.

To find the correct hand position, find the notch at the lower end of the victim's breastbone where the ribs meet the breastbone. Place the heel of one hand above this notch. Place your other hand directly on top of it. Try to keep your fingers off the chest by

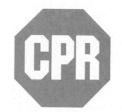

When to stop CPR

If another trained person takes over CPR for you.

If EMS personnel arrive and take over care of the victim.

If you are exhausted and unable to continue.

If the scene becomes unsafe.

The Shock of Your Life

Every year, 300,000 to 400,000 Americans collapse in their homes, in workplaces, or on the streets as a result of cardiac arrest. Ninety-five percent do not survive, but a simple, new, computerized device offers an increased chance for survival.

In two thirds of all cardiac arrests the heartbeat flutters wildly before it stops. The electric signals that tell the heart muscle to beat stops making sense. The heart is unable to send enough blood through the body. This condition is called ventricular fibrillation and can only be corrected by an electric shock.

Devices that could shock the heart into pumping effectively began to appear in 1966. These devices, called defibrillators, allowed medical personnel, away from the hospital, to monitor the heart's electrical activity. A doctor attached electrodes to the victim's chest to determine the heart's rhythm. If necessary, medical personnel delivered an electric shock to the heart to try to restore the heart's proper rhythm. In addition to doctors, paramedics eventually began to evaluate rhythms and deliver shocks at the emergency scene. Because of the expense and the lack of trained personnel across the United States, victims were not always able to get the lifesaving help that they needed.

Today a new, easy-to-use Automatic External Defibrillator (AED) allows emergency personnel and even citizen responders to provide the lifesaving shocks. The new defibrillators use a computer chip, rather than a medical professional, to analyze the heart's rhythm and deliver a shock if necessary. Typically, the user places two electrodes on the victim's chest. First the user presses the "Analyze" button, then, if the machine prompts the

user, he or she presses the "Shock" button. The machine does the rest.

Many first responders, like fire fighters and police officers, are trained to use AEDs. They can reduce the amount of time it takes to give a shock in a cardiac emergency because they are often the first people on the scene. By training the first responders, communities increase the number of emergency

personnel trained to use AEDs. In Eugene and Springfield, Oregon, authorities placed AEDs on every fire truck and trained all fire fighters to use them. The survival rates for cardiac arrest in these communities increased by 18 percent in the first year.

More than half of the states recognize defibrillator training for emergency medical technicians (EMTs). Author-

ities are also placing AEDs in areas where large groups of people gather, such as convention centers, stadiums, large businesses, and industrial complexes. Some experts hope that eventually AEDs will be as commonplace as fire alarms.

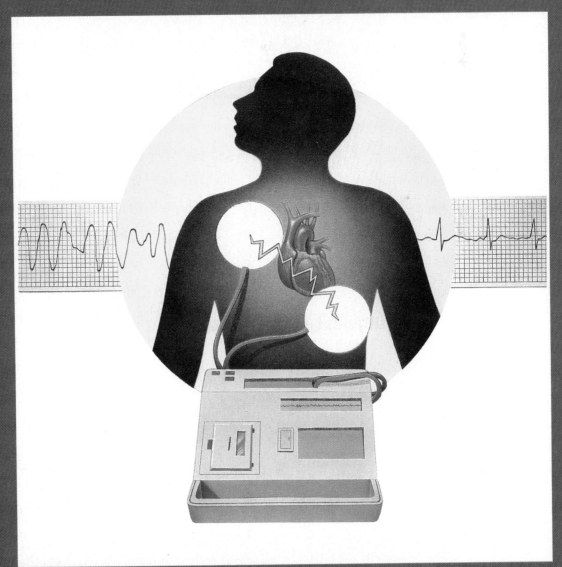

To find hand position, find the notch where the lower ribs meet the breastbone *(top)*. Place the heel of your hand on the breastbone, next to your index finger *(middle)*. Place your other hand on top of the first. Use the heel of your bottom hand to apply pressure on the breastbone *(bottom)*.

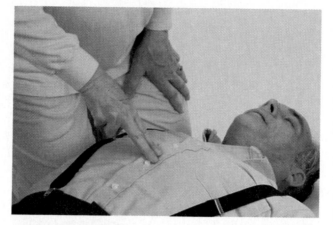

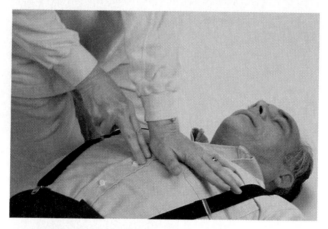

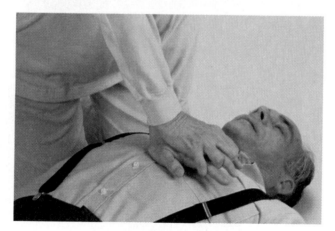

twining them together or sticking them out. If you have arthritis or a similar condition in your hands or wrists, you can give compressions while grasping the wrist of the hand positioned on the chest with your other hand.

Compress the chest by pressing down. Then release. You give chest compressions straight down in a smooth, even rhythm. Keep your shoulders directly over your hands and your elbows locked. Locking your elbows keeps your arms straight and prevents you from tiring quickly.

When you press down, the weight of your upper body creates the force you need to compress the chest. Push with the weight of your upper body, not with your arm muscles. Push straight down; don't rock. Each compression should push the chest down about 2 inches. After each compression, release the pressure on the chest without letting your hands lose contact with the chest. Allow the chest to return to its normal position before you give the next compression.

Keep a steady down-and-up rhythm and don't pause between compressions. Spend half the time going down and half coming up. If your hands slip, find the correct position again. Try not to move them off the chest or change their position.

As you do compressions, count "one and two and three and four and five and six and. . ." You should do 15 compressions in about 10 seconds. That's a little more than one compression per second.

Give 15 compressions, then retilt the head, lift the chin, and give 2 slow breaths. This cycle of 15 compressions and 2 breaths takes about 15 seconds.

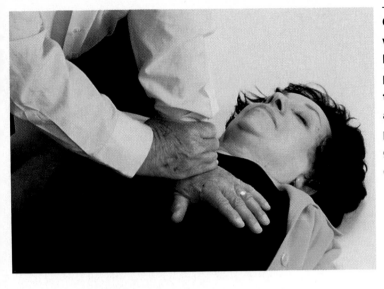

Grasping the wrist of the hand positioned on the chest is an alternate hand position for giving chest compressions.

Do four continuous cycles of CPR, which should take about 1 minute. Check the pulse at the end of the fourth cycle. If there is still no pulse, continue CPR. Check the pulse again every few minutes. If you find a pulse, check the victim's breathing. Give rescue breathing if necessary. If the victim is breathing, keep the head tilted back and check breathing and pulse until an ambulance arrives.

If another person at the scene says he or she knows how to do CPR, one of you should call for an ambulance while the other gives CPR. Then one of you can take over when the other one gets tired. To do this, the first rescuer stops at the end of a cycle of 15 compressions

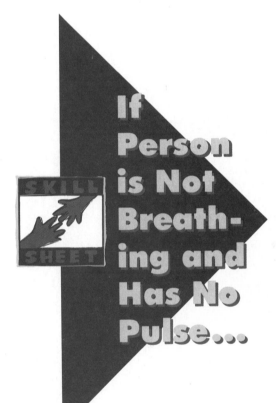

If Person is Not Breath-ing and Has No Pulse...

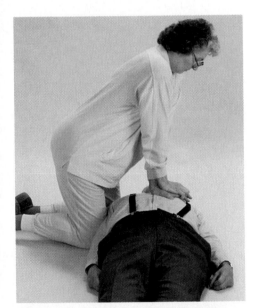

With your hands in place, position yourself so that your shoulders are directly over your hands and your elbows are locked. Press the chest down and then release it, keeping a smooth, even rhythm.

Give CPR

The emergency number has been called. If, when you check, the person is not breathing and has no pulse. . .

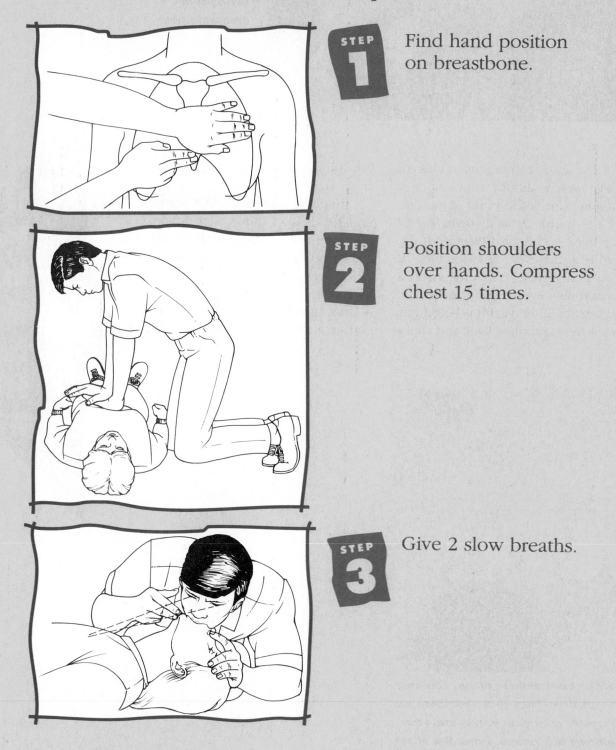

STEP 1
Find hand position on breastbone.

STEP 2
Position shoulders over hands. Compress chest 15 times.

STEP 3
Give 2 slow breaths.

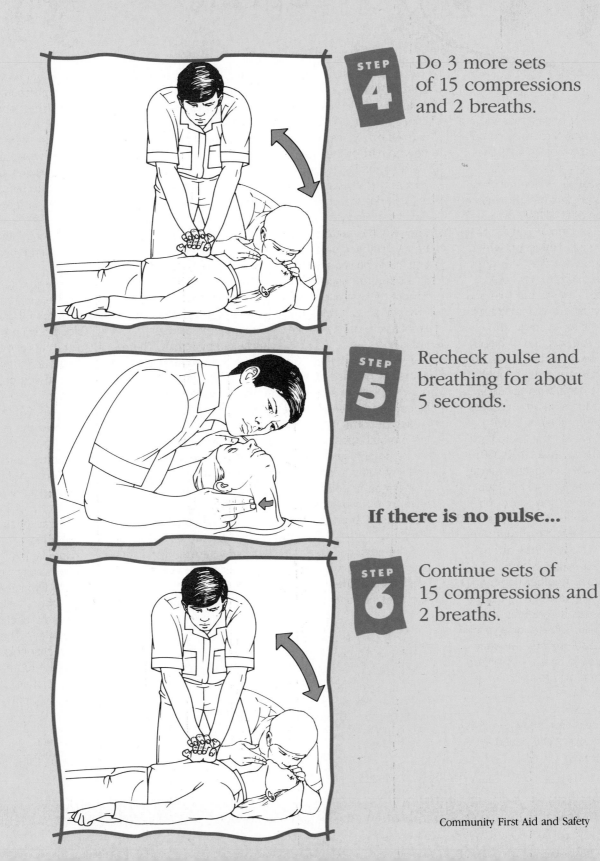

STEP 4 — Do 3 more sets of 15 compressions and 2 breaths.

STEP 5 — Recheck pulse and breathing for about 5 seconds.

If there is no pulse...

STEP 6 — Continue sets of 15 compressions and 2 breaths.

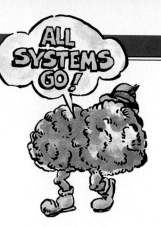

The Brain Speaks

Our brains speak to our bodies through a complex system of nerves, cells, and chemicals. In a healthy, well-functioning body this communication process allows us to swim, enjoy music, or tell a joke. However, when the brain does not get enough oxygen to its cells, some may die and cause brain damage, paralysis, or even death.

A disruption of blood flow to a part of the brain that is serious enough to damage brain tissue is called a stroke or a cerebrovascular accident (CVA). In the United States, about 150,000 people die each year because of strokes. Most are over the age of 65.

Stroke is usually caused by a blood clot that forms or lodges in the arteries that supply blood to the brain. Another common cause is bleeding from a damaged artery in the brain. A head injury, high blood pressure, a weak area in an artery wall, or fat deposits lining an artery may cause stroke. A tumor or swelling from a head injury may compress an artery and cause a stroke.

A transient ischemic attack (TIA) is sometimes called a "mini-stroke." Like a stroke, a TIA is caused by reduced blood flow to part of the brain. Unlike a stroke, the signals of a TIA disappear shortly, but the person is not out of danger. Someone who has a TIA has a nearly 10 times greater chance of having a stroke in the future. Since you cannot tell a stroke from a TIA, you should call for an ambulance for any stroke-like signals.

If you suspect that someone has had a stroke or a TIA, call for an ambulance immediately. If there is fluid or vomit in the victim's mouth, position him or her on one side to allow any fluids to drain out of the mouth. You may have to remove some of the material from the mouth.

If the person is conscious, offer comfort and reassurance. Often he or she does not understand

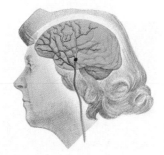

what has happened. Have the person rest in a comfortable position. Do not give the person anything to eat or drink. If the victim is drooling or having trouble swallowing, place him or her on one side to help drain any fluid from the mouth.

Ten years ago, a stroke almost always caused permanent brain damage. Today, new drugs and medical procedures can limit or, in some cases, reduce the damage caused by stroke. Therefore the sooner you call for an ambulance, the better the victim's chances are for a good recovery.

Preventing Stroke

Risk factors for stroke and TIA are similar to those for heart disease. Some risk factors are beyond your control, such as age, gender, or family history of stroke, TIA, diabetes, or heart disease.

You can control other risk factors. Most impor-

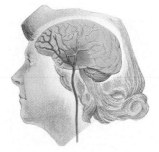

tant, if you have high blood pressure, talk with your doctor about ways to keep it down. High blood pressure increases your risk of stroke about seven times. High blood pressure puts pressure on arteries and makes them more likely to burst. Even mild high blood pressure can increase your risk of stroke.

Cigarette smoking is another major risk factor for stroke. It increases blood pressure and makes blood more likely to clot. If you don't smoke, don't start. If you do, get help to stop.

A diet high in saturated fats and cholesterol increases your chance of stroke by increasing the possibility of fatty materials building up on the walls of your blood vessels. Eat these foods in moderation.

Regular exercise reduces your chances of stroke by increasing blood circulation, which develops more channels for blood flow. These additional channels provide alternate routes for blood if the primary channels become blocked.

REFERENCE
National Safety Council. *Accident Facts*. Chicago, IL, 1991.

and 2 breaths. The second rescuer checks for breathing and pulse. If there is still no pulse, the second rescuer continues CPR.

Preventing Heart Disease

Recognizing a heart attack and getting the necessary care at once may prevent a victim from going into cardiac arrest. However, preventing a heart attack in the first place is even more effective. There is no substitute for prevention. Heart attacks are usually the result of disease of the heart and blood vessels. Heart disease is the leading cause of death for adults in the United States. It accounts for nearly 1 million deaths each year.

Heart disease develops slowly. Deposits of cholesterol, a fatty substance made by the body and present in certain foods, build up on the inner walls of the arteries. The arteries gradually narrow. As the arteries that carry blood to the heart get narrower, less oxygen-rich blood flows to the heart. This reduced oxygen supply to the heart can eventually cause a heart attack. When arteries in the brain narrow, a stroke can result.

Although a heart attack may seem to strike suddenly, many people live lives that are gradually putting their hearts in danger from heart disease. Because heart disease develops slowly, victims may not be aware of it for many years. Fortunately, it is possible to slow the progress of heart disease by making life-style changes.

Behavior that can harm the heart and blood vessels may begin in early childhood. We may develop a taste for "junk food," which is high in cholesterol but has little

Arteries of the heart

The arteries of the heart supply the heart muscle with blood. A buildup of materials on the inner walls of these arteries reduces the flow of oxygen-rich blood to the heart muscle, causing part of the heart to die. This is called a heart attack.

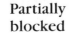

Unblocked

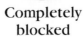

Partially blocked   Completely blocked

real food value. Heart disease can begin in the teens if those are the years when people begin to smoke. Smoking contributes to heart disease and to other diseases.

Many things increase a person's chances of developing heart disease. These are called risk factors. Some of them you can't change. For instance, men have a higher risk of heart disease than women. A history of heart disease in your family also increases your risk.

Many risk factors can be controlled, however. Smoking, eating a lot of fats, having high blood pressure, being overweight, and taking too little exercise all put you at greater risk of heart disease. When you combine one risk factor, like smoking, with others, such as high blood pressure and not enough exercise, your risk of heart attack or stroke is much greater.

People are becoming more aware of their risk factors for heart disease and are taking steps to control them. If you also take such steps, you will improve your chances for living a long and healthy life. Remember, it is never too late. Changes you make at any time in your life to lessen your risk will make a difference.

It is important to know how to do CPR. The truth remains, however, that the best way to deal with cardiac arrest is to prevent it. If you go into cardiac arrest, your chances of surviving are poor. Waiting to deal with cardiac arrest after it happens is like placing an ambulance at the bottom of a 100-foot cliff to be there when you fall off. Once you fall off the cliff, it's unlikely that even the best care can save your life. Preventing cardiac arrest, on the other hand, is like placing a barrier at the top of the cliff to keep you from tumbling to your death. Begin to reduce your risk of heart disease today.

Preventing Heart Disease

Heart disease is the leading cause of death for people over the age of 45 living in the United States. Although heart attacks may seem to strike suddenly, most of us make life-style choices every day that endanger our hearts. Over time, our choices can result in a heart attack or heart disease.

Scientists have identified factors that increase a person's chances of developing heart disease. These are known as risk factors. Some risk factors for heart disease cannot be changed. For example, men have a higher risk for heart disease than women. Having family members who have had heart disease also increases your risk.

Many risk factors for heart disease can be controlled. Smoking, diets high in fats, high blood pressure, obesity, and lack of routine exercise are all linked to increased risk of heart disease. When one risk factor, such as high blood pressure, is combined with other risk factors, the risk of heart attack or stroke is greatly increased. Managing your risk factors for heart disease really works. During the past 20 years, deaths from heart disease have gone down 33 percent in the United States, saving as many as 250,000 lives each year!

Smoking

Cigarette smokers have more than twice the chance of having a heart attack than non-smokers. They have two to four times the chance of cardiac arrest. The earlier a person starts smoking, the greater the risk to his or her health. Giving up smoking rapidly reduces the risk of heart disease. After a number of years, the risk for a person who stopped smoking is the same as the risk for a person who never smoked.

Recent studies indicate that even if you do not smoke, smoking may be increasing your risk of heart disease. Inhaling the smoke of others, called second-hand smoke, may be as dangerous as smoking. You should avoid long-term exposure to high levels of smoke and protect children from this potential danger. If you do not smoke, do not start. If you do smoke, quit.

Diet

Diets high in saturated fats and cholesterol increase the risk of heart disease. These diets raise the level of cholesterol found in the bloodstream. This increases the chances that cholesterol and other fatty deposits will be deposited on blood vessel walls, reducing blood flow.

Some cholesterol in the body is essential. The amount of cholesterol in the blood is determined by how much your body produces and by the food you eat. Foods high in cholesterol include egg yolks and organ meats such as liver, shrimp, and lobster.

A more significant contributor to an unhealthy blood-cholesterol level is saturated fat. Saturated fats raise the blood cholesterol level by interfering with the body's ability to remove cholesterol from the blood. Saturated fats are found in beef, lamb, veal, pork, ham, whole milk, and whole-milk products.

Rather than eliminating saturated fats and cholesterol from your diet, limit your intake. Moderation is the key. Make changes whenever possible. Substitute low fat or skimmed milk for whole milk and margarine for butter. Trim visible fat from meat and broil or bake instead of frying. Substitute fish for red meat occasionally. Eat fruit and vegetables for snacks instead of prepackaged or fast food. Read labels carefully. A "cholesterol free" product may actually be high in saturated fat.

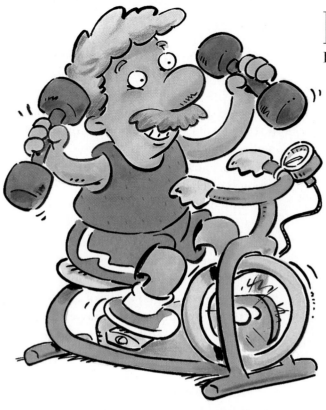

Exercise

Routine exercise has many benefits, including increased muscle tone and weight control. Exercise may also help you survive a heart attack because the increased circulation of blood through the heart develops additional channels for blood flow. If the primary channels that supply the heart are blocked in a heart attack, these additional channels can supply the heart with oxygen-rich blood.

Most of us wish we had more time to exercise. We know that exercise is good for almost every system in our body. But if you have limited time, it is best to build up cardiovascular fitness. Cardiovascular fitness can help you cope with stress, control your weight, ward off infections, improve self-esteem, sleep better, and accomplish your personal fitness goals.

To achieve cardiovascular fitness, you must exercise your heart. To do this, you should exercise at least three times a week for 20 to 30 minutes, maintaining your target heart rate range for at least 15 minutes. Your target heart rate range is 65 to 80 percent of your maximum heart rate. To find your target heart rate range, subtract your age from 220, then multiply that number by 0.65.

Consider a 40 year old who wants to exercise at 65 percent of his or her maximum heart rate. The target heart rate would be (220-40) x 0.65 = 117 beats per minute. This person should get his or her pulse rate to 117 beats per minute for at least 15 minutes during the workout.

As you exercise, take your pulse periodically at the wrist or neck. Exercise must be continuous and vigorous to maintain the target heart rate. As you build cardiovascular fitness, you will eventually be able to exercise for longer periods of time and at a higher target heart rate. The "no pain, no gain" theory is not a good approach to exercise. In fact, feeling pain usually means that you are exercising improperly. Be sure to warm up before vigorous exercise and cool down afterwards.

Turn your daily activities into exercise. Walk briskly or bicycle instead of driving. Climb the stairs instead of taking the elevator or escalator.

HEART HEALTHY IQ

HEALTH CHECK

The following statements represent a heart healthy life-style that can reduce your chances of heart disease. Check each statement that reflects your life-style.

- ☐ I do not smoke and I avoid inhaling the smoke of others.

- ☐ I eat a balanced diet that limits my intake of saturated fat and cholesterol.

- ☐ I participate in continuous, vigorous physical activity for 20 to 30 minutes or more at least three times a week.

- ☐ I have my blood pressure checked regularly.

- ☐ I maintain an appropriate weight.

If you did not check two or more of the statements, you should consider making changes in your life–style now.

Pedal an exercise bike or use a stair climber while watching TV, listening to music, or reading.

If you have not been exercising regularly or have health problems, see your doctor before starting an exercise program.

Blood Pressure

Uncontrolled high blood pressure can damage blood vessels in the heart and other organs. You can often control high blood pressure by losing excess weight and changing your diet. When these are not enough, a doctor can prescribe medications. You should take medications only as prescribed, and only your doctor should adjust them.

High blood pressure has no specific, easily recognized symptoms. It is important to have regular checkups to guard against high blood pressure and its effects. Free blood pressure checks may be available in your community at agencies, hospitals, health fairs, or pharmacies.

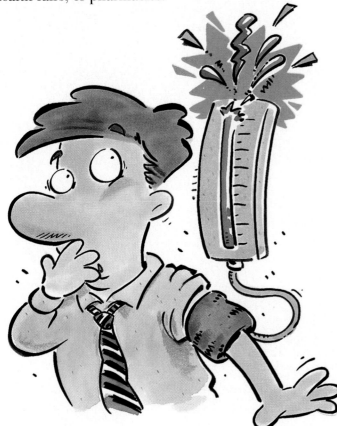

Weight

Many adults and children are overweight, some to the point of obesity. Obesity is defined as weighing 20 percent more than your desirable body weight. Obesity contributes to diseases such as heart disease, high blood pressure, diabetes, and gall bladder disease. However, body weight is not the main problem. The presence of too much body fat contributes to these diseases. See your doctor for help if you want a measure of your body fat.

Losing weight, especially fat, is no easy task. Weight loss and gain depend on a balance of intake of calories and output of energy. If you take in more calories than you use, you gain weight. If you use more calories that you take in, you lose weight.

Day-to-day weight changes reflect changes in the levels of fluids in your body. So if you are watching your weight, pick one day and time each week for your weigh-in. Track your weight loss based on this weekly amount, not on day-to-day differences.

Weight loss should always be combined with daily exercise. Any activity, such as walking to the bus, climbing the stairs, and cleaning the house, uses calories. The more active you are, the more calories you use.

Your eating habits should change as you grow older. If a person eats the same number of calories at the ages of 20 and 40 and maintains the same level of activity, he or she will be considerably heavier at 40 than at 20. It is important as you grow older to eat foods that provide your body with essential nutrients but are not high in calories.

When Seconds Count:

children

& Life-Threatening Emergencies

One in every 10 calls to your local EMS personnel is for an emergency involving children. If you are around children frequently, it is likely that you will have to care for a child or infant with an injury or illness. It is important to remember that children are not just small adults.

You might think that, because they are physically smaller, children do not need to breathe as fast as adults or that their hearts do not beat as fast.

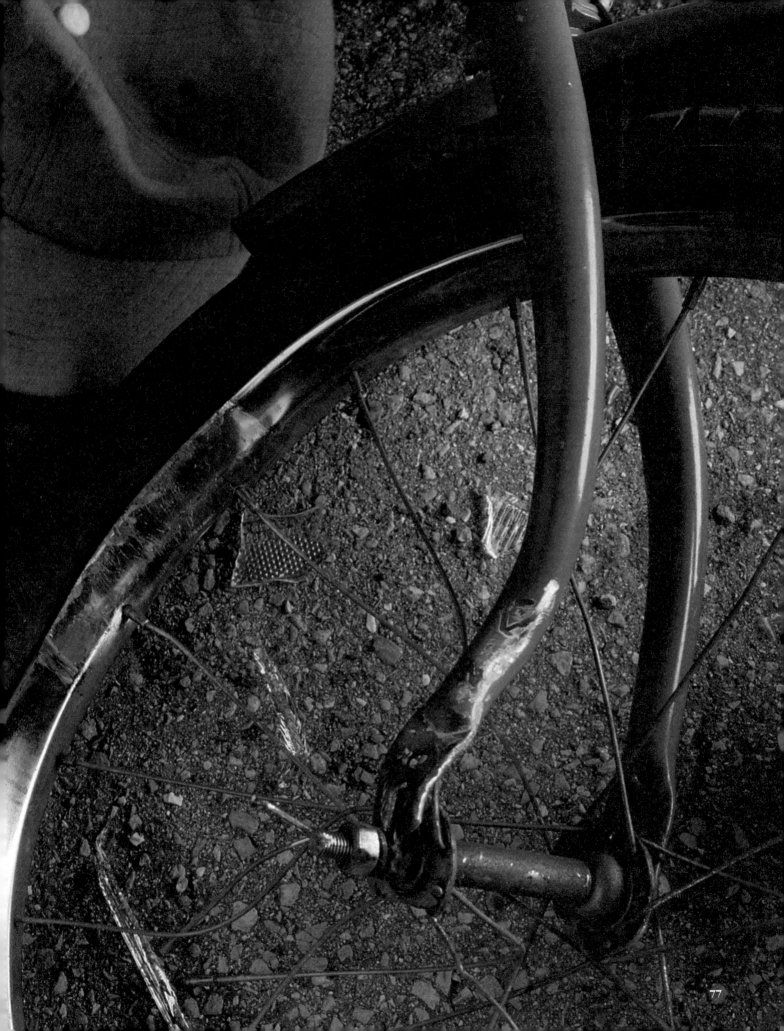

Injury...

is the leading cause of death of children in the U.S.

Children actually breathe faster than adults, and their hearts beat faster. The demands on their little bodies are great. In a breathing or cardiac emergency, children require care that is different from adults. Even among different-aged children, the care is somewhat different. Children from birth to 1 year of age receive slightly different care from that of children ages 1 to about 8.

In a life-threatening emergency, you must act at once. It may only be a matter of seconds before a child or infant dies. An emergency is life-threatening if the child or infant is unconscious, is not breathing, is breathing with difficulty, has no pulse, or is bleeding severely.

Let's take a look at the causes of life-threatening emergencies in children and infants. Before widespread immunization programs began about 40 years ago, infectious diseases, such as polio and diphtheria, were the main killers of chil-dren. Now injury is the leading cause of death in children in the United States. The numbers are staggering. Every year 600,000 children are admitted to a hospital with injuries.

The six most common types of childhood injuries are motor vehicle passenger injuries, pedestrian injuries, bicycle injuries, drowning, burns, and firearm injuries (including unintentional injuries, homicides, and suicides).

Most injuries can be prevented. If they were, childhood deaths and disabilities would be greatly reduced. As children grow and develop and as they are exposed to different environments, they become vulnerable to different injuries and illnesses. Adults have the responsibility of making the environment safe for children. This can be done by—

- Keeping children away from things that might harm them.

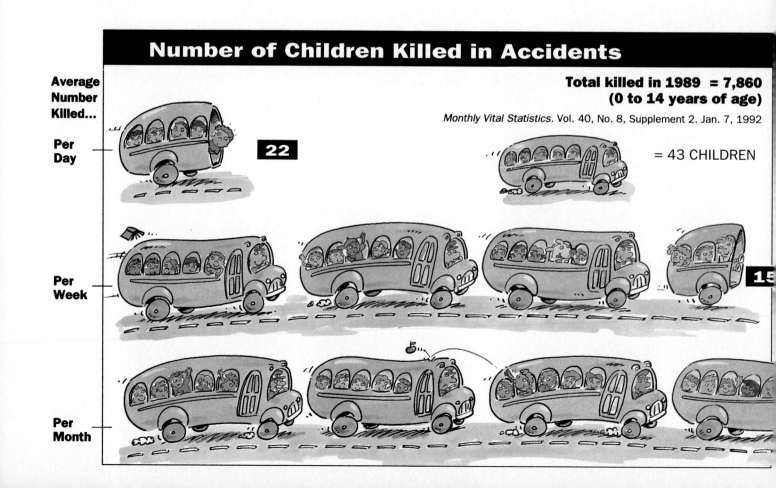

Number of Children Killed in Accidents

Average Number Killed...

Total killed in 1989 = 7,860
(0 to 14 years of age)

Monthly Vital Statistics. Vol. 40, No. 8, Supplement 2. Jan. 7, 1992

Per Day — 22   = 43 CHILDREN

Per Week — 15

Per Month

Why KIDS Always Get Hurt

Children are naturally curious about people and objects in the world around them. They spend much of their time exploring and learning. At the same time, their small bodies are growing quickly and becoming more mobile. A child's developing body, however, is less skilled and more prone to injury than an adult's. A child's body proportions are also different from an adult's. For example, a child's head is quite large and heavy compared with the rest of the body. This puts children at greater risk for head injuries. Children's eyesight and hearing take time to fully develop. Thus they are often injured by traffic that they don't hear or see while walking or cycling.

One way infants learn about their world is by putting objects in their mouths. They also grasp and pull with their hands and wiggle and move their bodies. All of these actions can lead them into danger. The infant who can pick up a button or coin can put it in his or her mouth and choke. The infant who can pull a cup from a coffee table can be burned by hot liquid. The infant who can roll over can roll off a bed and suffer a head injury. Infants face many new dangers as they learn to roll, crawl, stand, climb, and walk. Infants cannot recognize dangers and it is up to adults to protect them. Often, protecting them is as simple as removing the dangers. A bottle of furniture polish stored under a kitchen sink could poison a curious crawler. The danger can easily be removed by storing the polish in a locked cabinet where the child cannot reach it.

Like infants, toddlers and older children are always exploring and trying new things. Because they can walk, they tend to get into more trouble than infants do. They learn to copy adult behaviors and begin to understand how things work. They use words to ask for things and talk to other people, yet they lack judgment and understanding of potential risks. For instance, children cannot judge the depth of water.

Children are often injured when they are left alone, even for a few minutes. Young children need constant adult guidance and supervision, but the amount and kind of supervision needed changes as children grow and develop.

You can teach children safety in two ways. First, you can set an example of safe behavior by acting safely yourself. Second, you can encourage children to act safely by giving them simple, clear instructions about what they should and should not do. For example, teach children to always buckle their safety belts. Explain to them how a safety belt protects them from getting hurt. Teach them that they should not touch a hot stove and explain the meaning of the word *hot*. Remember to be patient. It takes time to learn safe behaviors and make them a habit.

> For more information on keeping children safe, contact:
>
> Consumer Product Safety Commission
> Washington, DC 20207
> **(800) 638-CPSC**
> Evaluates the safety of products sold to the public. Provides printed materials on consumer product safety topics on request.
>
> National Maternal and Child Health Clearinghouse
> 8201 Greensboro Drive, Suite 600
> McLean, VA 22102
> **(703) 821-8955, ext. 254**
> Provides information and printed materials on maternal and child health.

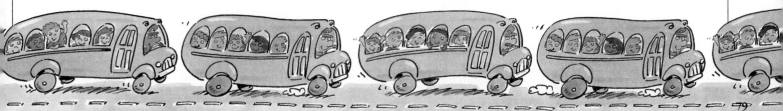

GENERAL SAFETY RULES

Here are some basic safety rules you can follow to protect children:

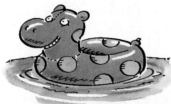

Buckle up children in motor vehicles.

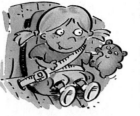

Always watch children in or near water.

Never keep loaded guns in your home.

Use gates on stairs.

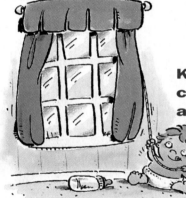

Keep plastic bags, cords, and small objects away from young children.

Call the Poison Control Center if you think a child has been poisoned.

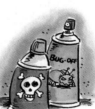

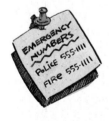

Have a plan for dealing with emergencies.

Check your home for fire and burn dangers.

- Staying near children so you can act in case of an emergency.
- Following safety rules yourself and teaching them to children.

Breathing Emergencies

The human body needs a constant supply of oxygen to stay alive. During breathing, air enters the nose and mouth. The air travels down the throat, through the windpipe, and into the lungs. This pathway from the nose and mouth to the lungs is called the airway. As you might well imagine, a child's airway is much smaller than an adult's. But as for an adult, the airway must be open for air to go into the lungs. In the lungs the oxygen in the air is picked up by the blood. The heart pumps the blood through the body. The blood flows through the blood vessels, taking the oxygen to the brain and to all other parts of the body.

A breathing emergency happens when air cannot travel freely and easily into the lungs. Some emergencies are life-threatening because they greatly cut down on the oxygen the body needs or cut off the oxygen entirely. For example, the body's supply of oxygen may be cut down when someone has difficulty breathing. However, when breathing stops, the oxygen supply is completely cut off. The heart will soon stop beating and blood will no longer move through the body. Unless the brain gets oxygen within minutes, brain damage or death will occur.

A breathing problem so severe that it threatens the victim's life is a breathing emergency. It is very im-

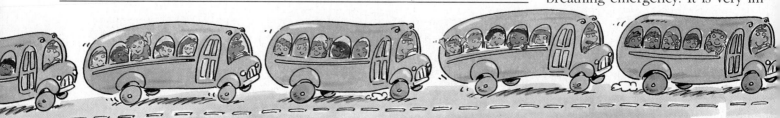

portant to recognize breathing emergencies in children and infants and to act before the heart stops beating. This is often the key to saving a child or infant's life.

Adult hearts frequently stop beating because they are diseased. For example, heart attacks are a common result of heart disease. Children's hearts, however, are usually healthy. When a child's heart stops, it is usually the result of a breathing emergency. If the child cannot breathe properly, not enough oxygen gets into the blood. This starves the heart of oxygen, and the heart soon stops beating. Children whose hearts stop beating rarely survive. Of the few who do, most suffer permanent brain damage.

Most cardiac emergencies in children can be prevented. There are three main ways to do this. One way is to keep children from being injured. A second is to make sure children have proper medical care. A third is to learn to recognize the early signals of a breathing emergency and what to do about such an emergency.

Breathing emergencies can be caused by injury or illness. Injury or disease in areas of the brain that control breathing can disturb or stop breathing. A major cause of breathing emergencies is choking on a piece of food or a small object.

Damage to the muscles or bones of the chest can make breathing painful or difficult. Electric shock and drowning can cause

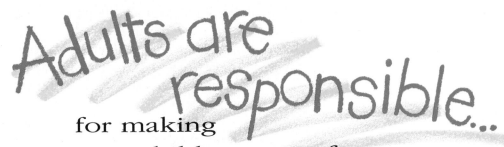

Adults are responsible... for making sure children are safe.

Air travels to the lungs by way of the airway, where oxygen is transferred to the blood. Oxygen-rich blood is transported to the brain, heart, and other parts of the body by way of the arteries.

655

breathing to stop. Allergic reactions may make the airway swell shut. Reactions to poisons, anxiety, excitement, and conditions such as asthma can all cause breathing emergencies.

Asthma is a condition that narrows the air passages and makes breathing difficult. It may be triggered by an allergic reaction to food, pollen, medications, bites, or stings or by physical or emotional stress. A typical signal of asthma is wheezing when the child breathes out. A child's chest may look larger than normal because air becomes trapped in the lungs. Normally, asthma is controlled with medication. Medications open the airway and make breathing easier.

Hyperventilation occurs when a child breathes faster than normal. Causes include fear or anxiety, injuries, illnesses such as high fever, and diabetic emergencies. It can also result from asthma or exercise. A typical signal of hyperventilation is shallow, rapid breathing. Despite trying hard to breathe, children who are hyperventilating say they

Unless the brain gets oxygen...

brain damage or death will occur within minutes.

SIGNALS OF A BREATHING EMERGENCY

CHECK BREATHING
Breathing is—
Slower or faster than usual.
Noisy.
Painful.

Child or infant is—
Gasping for breath.
Wheezing, gurgling, or making high-pitched sounds.

CHECK SKIN
Skin is more moist than usual.
Skin looks flushed, pale, or bluish.

ASK HOW CHILD FEELS
Child feels—
Short of breath.
Dizzy or light-headed.
Pain in the chest.
Tingling in the hands and feet.

If you see any signals of a breathing emergency, you should get medical care at once!

cannot get enough air or that they are suffocating. Therefore they are often frightened and confused. They may say that they feel dizzy or that their fingers and toes feel numb or tingly.

A severe allergic reaction can cause the airway to swell and restrict breathing. It may result from insect stings, food, or medications, such as penicillin. If you know a child is allergic to certain substances, keep the child away from them. A physician may recommend that the child or an adult guardian carry medication to reverse the reaction.

Signals of allergic reaction may develop very quickly. They include a rash, a feeling of tightness in the chest and throat, and swelling of the face, neck, and tongue. The child may feel dizzy or confused. If not cared for at once, severe allergic reactions can become life-threatening.

Even though there are many causes of breathing emergencies, you don't have to know the exact cause to respond. You do need to be able to recognize the signals of a breathing emergency and take action fast!

Recognizing Breathing Emergencies

You are most likely to have to care for a conscious child or infant who is having difficulty breathing. You will probably be able to identify a breathing problem by watching and listening to the way the child or infant breathes. A child who can talk may be able to tell you what is wrong.

Normal breathing is easy and quiet. Children should not have to work at breathing. Breaths should be regular, and breathing should not be painful.

When a child's heart stops...

it is usually the result of a breathing emergency.

There are many signals of breathing emergencies. They might not be the same for all children. Children and infants may look as if they can't catch their breath, or they may gasp for air. They may be breathing faster or slower than normal. Their breaths may be deeper or more shallow than usual. They may make unusual noises, such as wheezing or gurgling, or high-pitched sounds.

The child's skin may also signal that something is wrong. At first, the child's skin may be more moist than usual and look flushed. Later, it may look pale or bluish as the oxygen level in the blood falls.

A child having a breathing problem may feel dizzy or light-headed. The child may complain that his or her chest hurts and that his or her hands and feet are tingling. The child may be frightened.

Any of these signals indicates a breathing emergency. In short, any breathing that is noisy, painful, or unusually fast or slow is a breathing emergency.

A child who can talk may be able to tell you that he or she finds it difficult to breathe. For infants and very young children, though, you must use your own judgment based on how the child looks and the way he or she is breathing. If you see any signals of a breathing emergency, you should get medical care at once.

Make Your Home Safe for Kids

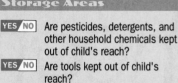

Storage Areas

YES/NO Are pesticides, detergents, and other household chemicals kept out of child's reach?

YES/NO Are tools kept out of child's reach?

General Safety Precautions Inside the Home

YES/NO Are stairways kept clear and uncluttered?

YES/NO Are stairs and hallways well lit?

YES/NO Are safety gates installed at tops and bottoms of stairways?

YES/NO Are guards installed around fireplaces, radiators or hot pipes, and wood-burning stoves?

YES/NO Are sharp edges of furniture cushioned with corner guards or other material?

YES/NO Are unused electric outlets covered with tape or safety covers?

YES/NO Are curtain cords and shade pulls kept out of child's reach?

YES/NO Are windows secured with window locks?

YES/NO Are plastic bags kept out of child's reach?

YES/NO Are fire extinguishers installed where they are most likely to be needed?

YES/NO Are smoke detectors in working order?

YES/NO Do you have an emergency plan to use in case of fire? Does your family practice this plan?

YES/NO Is the water set at a safe temperature? (A setting of 120° F or less prevents scalding from tap water in sinks and in tubs. Let the water run for three minutes before testing it.)

YES/NO If you have a gun, is it locked in a place where your child cannot get it?

YES/NO Are all purses, handbags, brief cases, and so on, including those of visitors, kept out of child's reach?

YES/NO Are all poisonous plants kept out of child's reach?

YES/NO Is a list of emergency phone numbers posted near a telephone?

YES/NO Is a list of instructions posted near a telephone for use by children and/or babysitters?

Bathroom

YES/NO Are the toilet seat and lid kept down when the toilet is not in use?

YES/NO Are cabinets equipped with safety latches and kept closed?

YES/NO Are all medicines in child-resistant containers and stored in a locked medicine cabinet?

YES/NO Are shampoos and cosmetics stored out of child's reach?

YES/NO Are razors, razor blades, and other sharp objects kept out of child's reach?

YES/NO Are hair dryers and other appliances stored away from sink, tub, and toilet?

YES/NO Does the bottom of tub or shower have rubber stickers or a rubber mat to prevent slipping?

YES/NO Is the child always watched by an adult while in the tub?

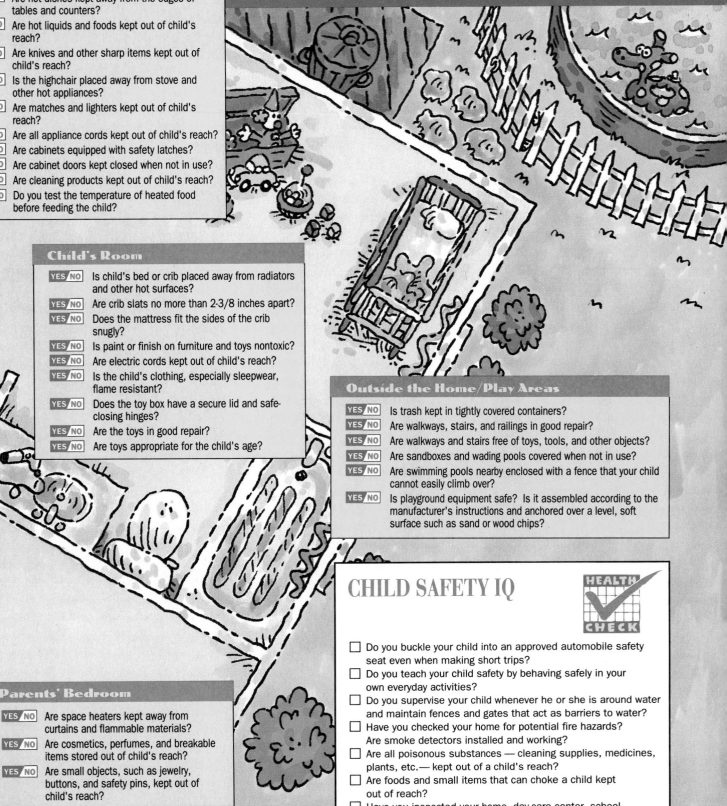

Kitchen

- YES/NO Do you cook on back stove burners when possible and turn pot handles toward the back of the stove?
- YES/NO Are hot dishes kept away from the edges of tables and counters?
- YES/NO Are hot liquids and foods kept out of child's reach?
- YES/NO Are knives and other sharp items kept out of child's reach?
- YES/NO Is the highchair placed away from stove and other hot appliances?
- YES/NO Are matches and lighters kept out of child's reach?
- YES/NO Are all appliance cords kept out of child's reach?
- YES/NO Are cabinets equipped with safety latches?
- YES/NO Are cabinet doors kept closed when not in use?
- YES/NO Are cleaning products kept out of child's reach?
- YES/NO Do you test the temperature of heated food before feeding the child?

Use this checklist to spot dangers in your home. When you read each question, circle either the "Yes" box or the "No" box. Each "No" shows a possible danger for you and your family. Work with your family to remove dangers and make your home safer.

Child's Room

- YES/NO Is child's bed or crib placed away from radiators and other hot surfaces?
- YES/NO Are crib slats no more than 2-3/8 inches apart?
- YES/NO Does the mattress fit the sides of the crib snugly?
- YES/NO Is paint or finish on furniture and toys nontoxic?
- YES/NO Are electric cords kept out of child's reach?
- YES/NO Is the child's clothing, especially sleepwear, flame resistant?
- YES/NO Does the toy box have a secure lid and safe-closing hinges?
- YES/NO Are the toys in good repair?
- YES/NO Are toys appropriate for the child's age?

Outside the Home/Play Areas

- YES/NO Is trash kept in tightly covered containers?
- YES/NO Are walkways, stairs, and railings in good repair?
- YES/NO Are walkways and stairs free of toys, tools, and other objects?
- YES/NO Are sandboxes and wading pools covered when not in use?
- YES/NO Are swimming pools nearby enclosed with a fence that your child cannot easily climb over?
- YES/NO Is playground equipment safe? Is it assembled according to the manufacturer's instructions and anchored over a level, soft surface such as sand or wood chips?

Parents' Bedroom

- YES/NO Are space heaters kept away from curtains and flammable materials?
- YES/NO Are cosmetics, perfumes, and breakable items stored out of child's reach?
- YES/NO Are small objects, such as jewelry, buttons, and safety pins, kept out of child's reach?

CHILD SAFETY IQ

HEALTH CHECK

- ☐ Do you buckle your child into an approved automobile safety seat even when making short trips?
- ☐ Do you teach your child safety by behaving safely in your own everyday activities?
- ☐ Do you supervise your child whenever he or she is around water and maintain fences and gates that act as barriers to water?
- ☐ Have you checked your home for potential fire hazards? Are smoke detectors installed and working?
- ☐ Are all poisonous substances — cleaning supplies, medicines, plants, etc.— kept out of a child's reach?
- ☐ Are foods and small items that can choke a child kept out of reach?
- ☐ Have you inspected your home, day-care center, school, babysitter's home, or wherever your child spends time for potential safety and health hazards?
- ☐ Do you keep guns and ammunition stored separately and locked up?

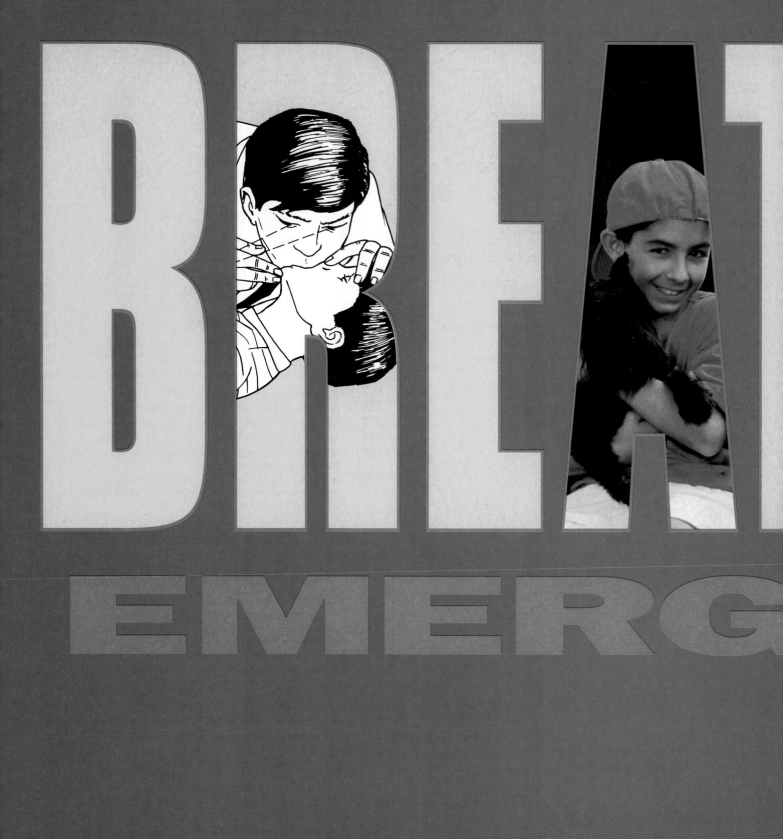

CARING FOR

BREA

EMERG

CHILDREN WITH

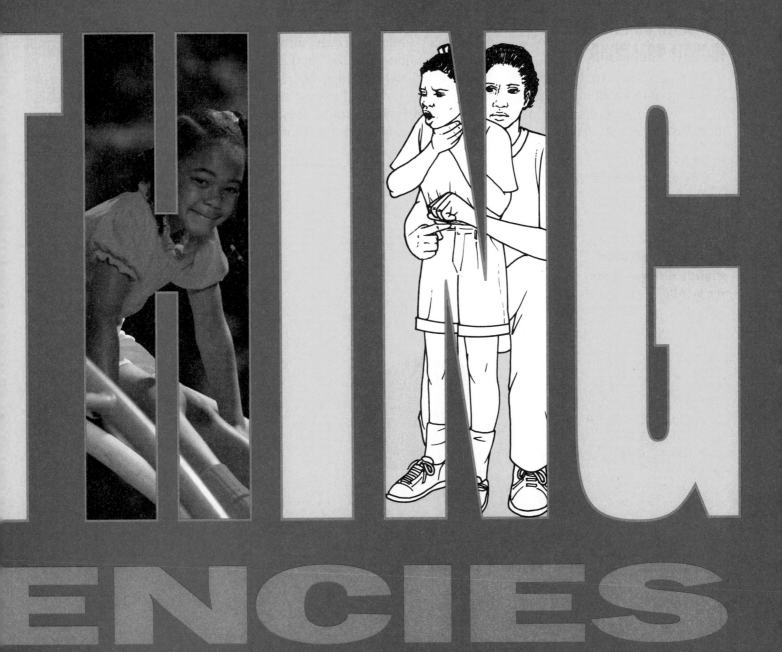

THING
ENCIES

Recognizing the signals of breathing emergencies and caring for them are often keys to preventing other emergencies. A breathing problem may signal the beginning of a life-threatening condition.

IF A CHILD OR INFANT HAS TROUBLE BREATHING

If a conscious child or infant is having trouble breathing, help him or her rest in a comfortable position. Sitting usually makes breathing easier. Make sure someone has called the local emergency number for help. Stay with the child or infant until an ambulance arrives.

Remember that children who are having difficulty breathing may have trouble talking. Talk to any bystanders who may know the child's problem. Children often answer yes-or-no questions by nodding. Keep checking breathing and skin appearance. Try to reduce any anxiety that might have contributed to the breathing problem by comfort-

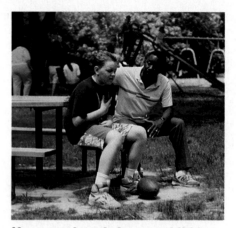

If a conscious infant or child is having trouble breathing, support him or her in a sitting position.

Care for an infant is slightly different than for a child.

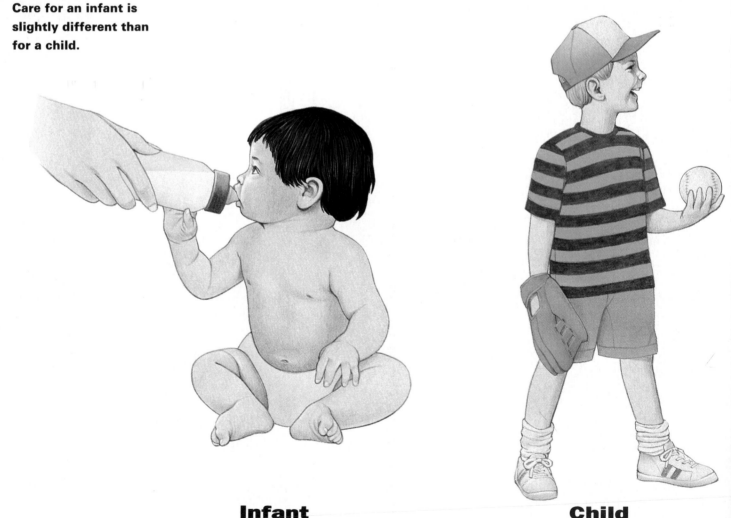

**Infant
(0-1 YEAR)**

**Child
(1-8 YEARS)**

ing him or her. Help keep the child or infant from getting chilled or overheated. Help give any medication prescribed for a particular condition.

If the child or infant is breathing rapidly (hyperventilating) and you are sure it is caused by emotion, such as excitement, not injury or illness, try to get the child to relax and breathe slowly. Reassurance is often enough to correct hyperventilation. If the child's breathing still does not return to normal or if the child becomes unconscious from hyperventilating, call the local emergency number right away.

If you recognize the signals of a breathing emergency and can provide care, you may be able to prevent the condition from developing into a more serious emergency. If the child stops breathing, he or she may die without immediate care.

The care for infants and for children with breathing emergencies is similar. But as you read earlier, some of the techniques are a little different because infants and children vary in size. In general, skills that are described for a child should be used for a child from about age 1 to about age 8. Infant skills should be used for those under 1 year of age. A general guideline is to perform infant skills on a child or infant about the length of your thigh or whom you can comfortably support with your forearm and hand. Perform child skills on a child who is larger than this.

CARING FOR BREATHING DIFFICULTY

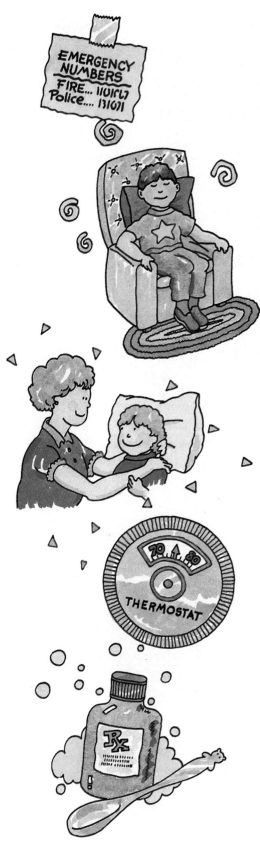

Call the local emergency phone number for help.

Help the child or infant rest in the position easiest for breathing.

Comfort the child or infant.

Keep checking breathing.

Make sure the child or infant does not get chilled or overheated.

Give any prescribed medication.

PREVENTING CHOKING

Don't leave small objects, such as buttons, coins, and beads, within an infant's reach.

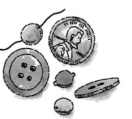

Have children sit in a high chair or at a table while they eat.

Do not let children eat too fast.

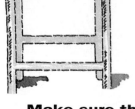

Give infants soft food that they do not need to chew.

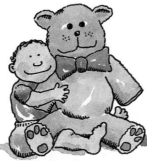

Make sure that toys are too large to be swallowed.

Do not give infants and young children foods like nuts, grapes, popcorn, and raw vegetables.

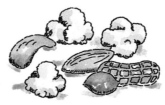

Make sure that toys have no small parts that could be pulled off.

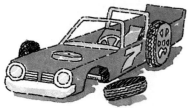

Cut foods a child can choke on easily, such as hot dogs, into small pieces.

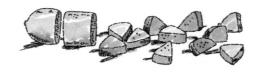

Supervise children while they eat.

IF A CHILD IS CHOKING

Choking is a common childhood injury that can lead to death. When a child is choking, the airway is partly or completely blocked, usually by food or other small objects. Children often choke while they are eating and can choke on a very small piece of food. Also, children cannot or do not always chew food well. Some foods that an adult can eat easily can cause a child to choke.

Tasting is one way children explore their world. Young children, especially those under the age of three, often put objects, such as coins, beads, and toys, in their mouths. This is normal, but it can lead to choking.

A choking child can quickly stop breathing, lose consciousness, and die. Therefore it is very impor-

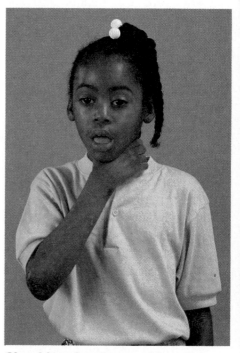

Clutching the throat with one or both hands is universally recognized as a distress signal for choking.

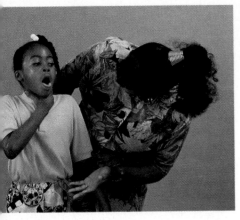

Encourage a choking child who is coughing forcefully to continue coughing.

tant to recognize when a child needs first aid for choking. One of the signals of choking is coughing. Sometimes a child who is choking will cough forcefully. At other times the child may cough weakly or make a high-pitched sound while coughing. A child who is not able to breathe or cough at all may panic and clutch his or her throat with one or both hands.

If the child is coughing forcefully, the airway is partially blocked but the child is still able to get some air. Stay with the child. Tell the child to keep on coughing. The coughing may clear the airway. If the child does not stop coughing soon or does not cough up the object, call the local emergency number for help.

If the child is coughing weakly or is making a high-pitched sound or if the child cannot speak, breathe, or cough, the airway is completely blocked. You must give first aid right away. Try to remove the object that is blocking the airway by creating an artificial cough. Wrap your arms around the child's waist. Make a fist with one hand and place it against the middle of the child's abdomen, just above the navel. Grab your fist with your other hand. Give quick upward thrusts into the abdomen until the object is forced out.

Stop giving thrusts as soon as the child coughs up the object or

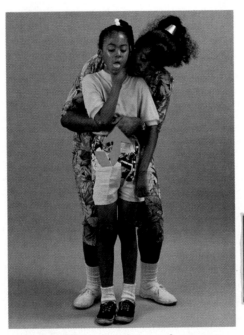

If a child is choking and cannot speak, give quick, upward thrusts to the abdomen, just above the navel, until the object is forced out.

starts to breathe or cough. Watch the child and make sure that he or she is breathing freely again. Even after the child coughs up the object, the child may have breathing problems that will need a doctor's attention. Also, abdominal thrusts may cause injuries. For these reasons, you should call the local emergency number if you have not already done so. The child should be taken to the hospital emergency department to be checked by a physician. Do this even if the child seems to be breathing well.

SKILL SHEET

If Child is Unable to Speak, Cough, or Breathe...

Give Abdominal Thrusts

If, when you check, the child is unable to speak, cough, cry, or breathe. . .

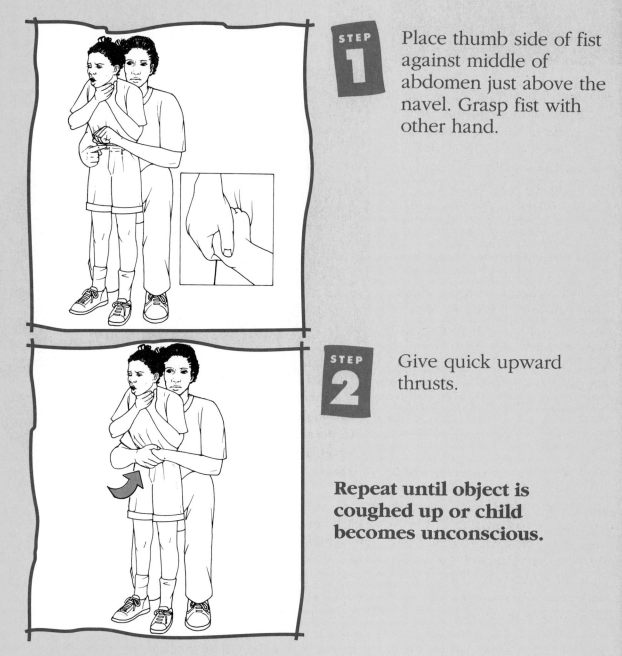

STEP 1 Place thumb side of fist against middle of abdomen just above the navel. Grasp fist with other hand.

STEP 2 Give quick upward thrusts.

Repeat until object is coughed up or child becomes unconscious.

IF A CHILD IS NOT BREATHING

A child may stop breathing because of illness, injury, or a blocked airway. A child who is not breathing gets no oxygen. The body can function only for a few minutes without oxygen before body systems begin to fail.

A child who is not breathing needs rescue breathing. Rescue breathing is a way of breathing air into a person to supply the oxygen he or she needs to survive. Rescue breathing is given to any child who is not breathing.

You discover whether you need to give rescue breathing when you check an unconscious child. If the child is not breathing but has a pulse, begin rescue breathing. Begin by tilting the head back and lifting the chin to move the tongue away from the back of the throat.

This opens the airway. Place your ear next to the child's mouth. Look, listen, and feel for breathing for about 5 seconds. If you can't see, hear, or feel any signs of breathing, pinch the child's nose shut and make a tight seal around the child's mouth with your mouth. Breathe slowly into the child until you see the chest rise. Do this two times. Each breath should last about 1½ seconds. Pause between each breath to let the air flow back out. Watch the child's chest rise each time you breathe into the child to be sure that your breaths are actually going in.

Check for a pulse at the side of the neck. If a pulse is present but the child is still not breathing, give 1 breath about every 3 seconds. A good way to time the breaths is to count "one one-thousand," take a breath on "two one-thousand" and

1 BREATH 3 SECONDS

If there is a pulse but the child is not breathing, give 1 breath about every 3 seconds.

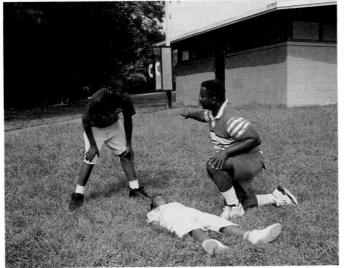

If someone is with you when you discover an unconscious child, have that person phone for help while you continue to give care.

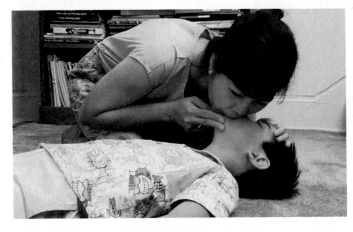

If a child stops breathing, you must breathe for him or her. This is called rescue breathing.

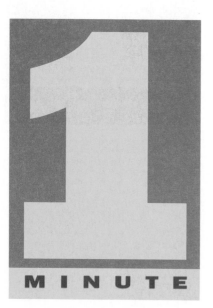

1
MINUTE

If you are alone and the child is not breathing, give rescue breathing for about 1 minute before calling your emergency number.

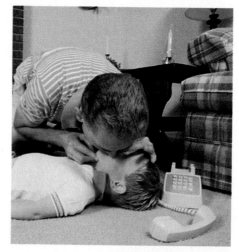

If the child is small enough, carry him or her to the phone while you continue to give breaths.

If vomiting occurs, turn the child on his or her side and wipe the mouth clean.

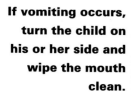

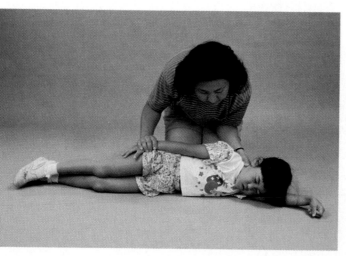

breathe into the child on "three one-thousand."

After about 1 minute of rescue breathing (about 20 breaths), re-check the pulse. If the child still has a pulse but is not breathing, continue rescue breathing. Check the pulse every minute. Continue rescue breathing until one of the following happens:

• The child begins to breathe on his or her own.
• The child has no pulse (begin CPR).
• Another trained rescuer takes over for you.
• You are too tired to go on.

Call the local emergency number for help if a child is unconscious. If someone is with you when you discover an unconscious child, have that person phone for help immediately. This way, you can continue checking the child and give rescue breathing or any other necessary care at once. If you are alone and you find a child unconscious and not breathing, give rescue breathing for about 1 minute before calling the local emergency number. This delay in phoning allows you to give breaths that will get oxygen into the child and prevent the heart from stopping. If the child is small enough, carry him or her to the telephone while continuing to give breaths.

When you are giving rescue breathing, you want to avoid getting air in the child's stomach instead of the lungs. This may happen if you breathe into the child too long, breathe too hard, or don't open the airway far enough.

To avoid getting air in the child's stomach, keep the child's head tilted back. Breathe *slowly* into the child, just enough to make the chest rise. Each breath should last about 1½ seconds. Pause between breaths long enough for the air in the child's lungs to come out and for you to take another breath.

Air in the stomach can make the child vomit. When an unconscious child vomits, the contents of the stomach can get into the lungs and block breathing. Air in the stomach also makes it harder for the diaphragm, the large muscle that controls breathing, to move. This makes it harder for the lungs to fill with air.

Even when you are giving rescue breathing properly, the child may vomit. If this happens, roll the child onto one side and wipe the mouth clean. If possible, use latex

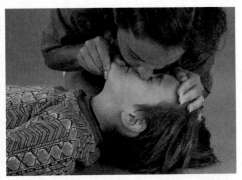

For mouth-to-nose breathing, close the child's mouth, seal your mouth around the child's nose, and breathe into the nose.

gloves, gauze, or even a handkerchief when you sweep out the mouth. Then roll the child on his or her back again and continue with rescue breathing.

Sometimes you might not be able to make a tight enough seal over a child's mouth. For example, the child's jaw or mouth may be injured or shut too tightly to open. If you can't make a tight seal over the mouth, you can breathe into the nose. With the head tilted backward, close the child's mouth by gently pushing on the chin. Seal your mouth around the child's nose and breathe into the nose. If possible, open the child's mouth between breaths to let the air out.

Finally, you should suspect head, neck, or back injuries if a child has fallen from a height or has been in a motor vehicle crash. If you suspect such an injury, try not to move the child's head and neck. If you need to open the airway, do so by lifting the child's chin without tilting the head back. This may be enough to allow air to pass into the lungs. If you try to give breaths and your breaths are not going in, you should tilt the head back very slightly. This will usually allow air to pass into the lungs. If air still does not go in, tilt the head farther back. It is unlikely that this action will make any injuries worse. Remember that if a child isn't breathing, his or her greatest need is for air.

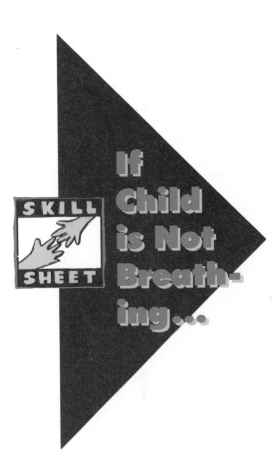

SKILL SHEET

If Child is Not Breathing...

If you suspect a head or spine injury, try to open the airway by lifting the chin without tilting the head.

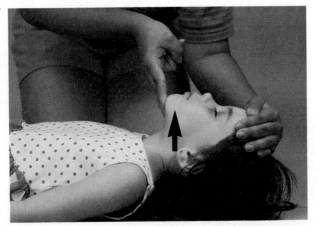

Give Rescue Breathing

The emergency number has been called. If, when you check, the child is not breathing. . .

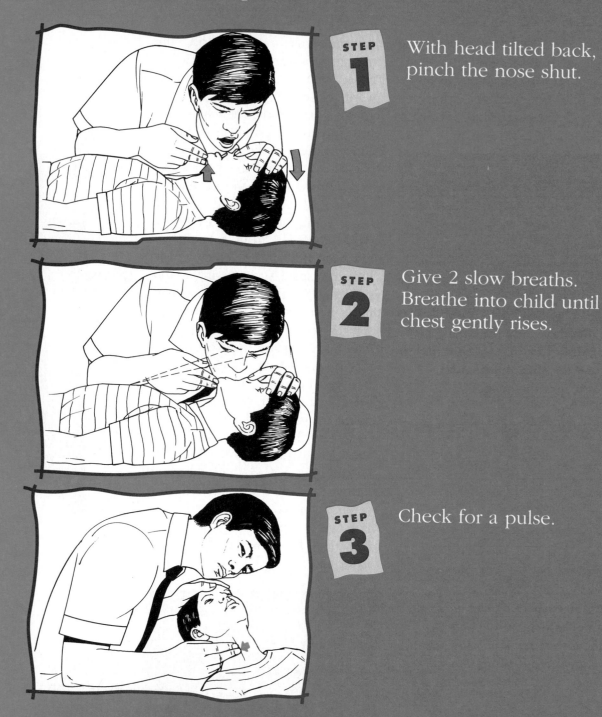

STEP 1
With head tilted back, pinch the nose shut.

STEP 2
Give 2 slow breaths. Breathe into child until chest gently rises.

STEP 3
Check for a pulse.

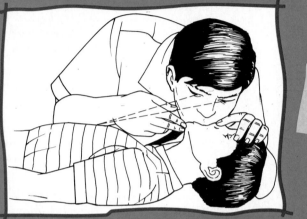

If a pulse is present but child is still not breathing ...

 STEP 4 Give 1 slow breath about every 3 seconds. Do this for about 1 minute (20 breaths).

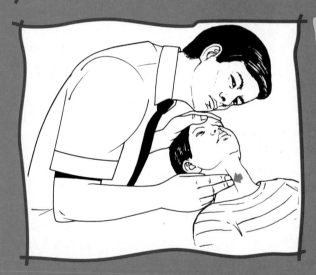

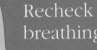 **STEP 5** Recheck pulse and breathing.

Call the local emergency number if you have not already done so. Then, continue rescue breathing as long as a pulse is present but child is not breathing.

Recheck pulse and breathing about every minute.

IF AIR WON'T GO IN

You may find that an unconscious child's chest does not rise and fall as you give breaths. If you did not tilt the head back far enough, the child's tongue may be blocking the throat. Retilt the child's head and give two more breaths. If you still cannot breathe air into the child, the child's airway is probably blocked. The airway can be blocked by food, a small object such as a toy or coin, or fluids such as blood and saliva. Tell someone to phone the local emergency number for help while you provide care.

The most important thing to do is to try to remove the object or move it enough so you can get air past it into the lungs. First, try to create an artificial cough to force air—and the object—out of the airway. To do this, press both hands into the child's abdomen with quick upward thrusts. To give thrusts, straddle the child. Place the heel of one hand on the middle of the abdomen just above the navel. Place the other hand on top of the first. Give thrusts toward the head. Give up to five thrusts, then look to see if the object is in the child's mouth. If you can see the object, slide a finger down the inside of the child's cheek and try to hook the object out. Next give two breaths.

If your first attempts to clear the airway don't succeed, repeat the abdominal thrusts, object checks, and breaths. The longer the child goes without oxygen, the more the muscles of the throat will relax. This will make it more likely you will be able to remove the object or breathe past it.

If you do clear the airway and can breathe into the child, give two slow breaths and check the child's pulse. If there is a pulse, check for breathing. If the child is not breathing on his or her own, continue rescue breathing.

If the child starts breathing on his or her own, keep the airway open and continue to check breathing until EMS personnel arrive and take over.

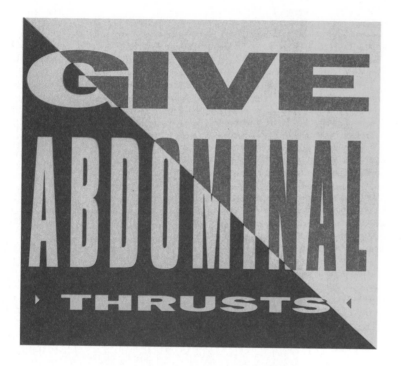

If you are unable to breathe air into the child, the airway is probably blocked. Give abdominal thrusts.

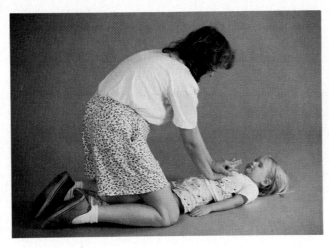

To give abdominal thrusts to a child, straddle the legs, position your hands with your fingers pointing toward the victim's head and give quick, upward thrusts.

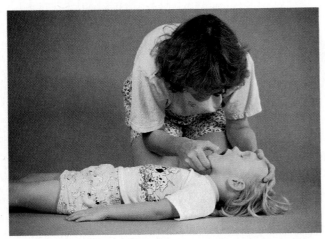

Look for an object in the throat. Slide a finger down inside of the cheek and try to hook the object out only if you can see it.

SKILL SHEET

If Air Does Not Go In...

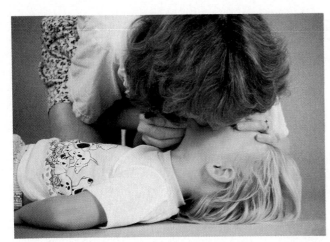

Open the airway and attempt to give 2 breaths.

The emergency number has been called. If, when you check, the child is not breathing and your breaths do not go in. . .

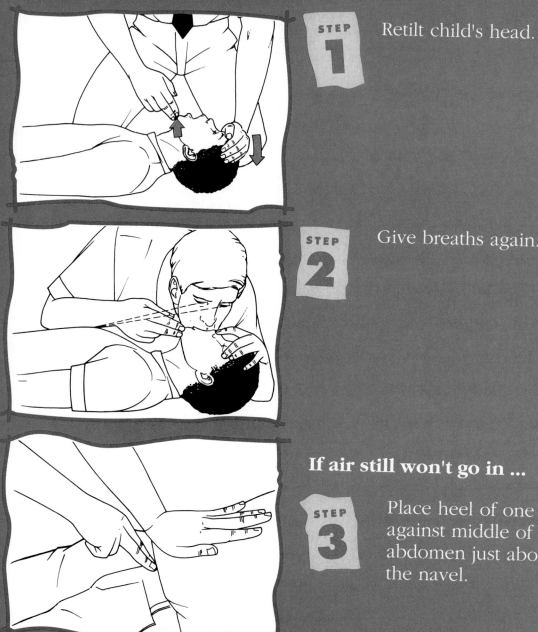

STEP 1 Retilt child's head.

STEP 2 Give breaths again.

If air still won't go in ...

STEP 3 Place heel of one hand against middle of abdomen just above the navel.

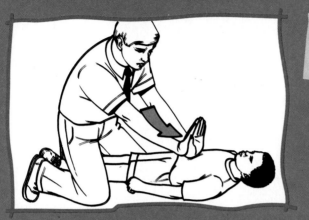

STEP 4

Give up to 5 abdominal thrusts.

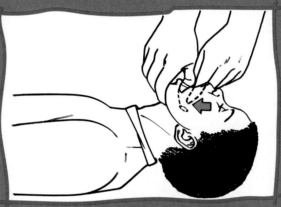

STEP 5

Lift jaw and tongue and check for object. If seen, sweep it out with finger.

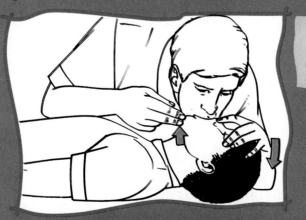

STEP 6

Tilt head back and give breaths again.

Repeat breaths, thrusts, and checks for object until breaths go in or child starts to breathe on own.

Call the local emergency number after giving care for 1 minute if you have not already done so.

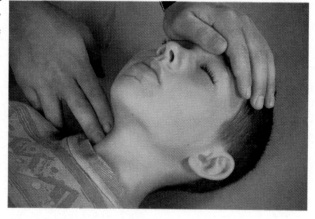

For a child, check for a pulse at the side of the neck.

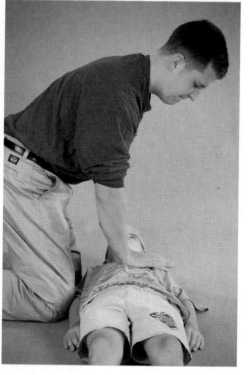

To give compressions, keep the head tilted back and place the heel of your other hand on the lower half of the breastbone. Press the chest down and then release it in a smooth, even rhythm.

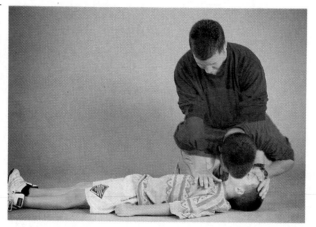

When giving CPR, alternate chest compressions and rescue breathing.

IF A CHILD DOES NOT HAVE A PULSE

Your check of an unconscious child includes checking breathing and pulse. If the child is not breathing, it is likely that his or her heart will stop beating. Checking the pulse can tell you whether or not the child's heart has stopped. For a child, check for a pulse at the side of the neck. If you can't feel the pulse after checking for about 5 to 10 seconds, you should start cardiopulmonary resuscitation (CPR).

CPR has two parts. One part is chest compressions. When you give chest compressions, press down and let up on the lower half of the breastbone. The second part of CPR is rescue breathing. When you give CPR, alternate chest compressions and rescue breathing.

When you breathe into the lungs of a child who has stopped breathing, you keep the lungs supplied with oxygen. The oxygen in the lungs goes into the blood. When you compress the chest, you keep blood flowing through the child's body. The blood carries oxygen to the brain, heart, and other parts of the body. CPR keeps oxygen-carrying blood flowing through the body, especially to the brain.

You must start CPR as soon as possible after the child's heart stops beating. If brain cells don't get oxygen, they begin to die after 4 minutes. Starting CPR right away increases the chances that the child will survive.

Once you have decided that the child needs CPR, you must put yourself and the child in the correct position. Place the child on his or her back, on a firm, level surface. Kneel beside the child's chest. Keep the child's head tilted back with one hand. Place your other

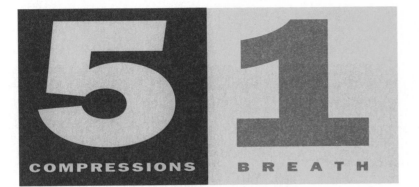

5 COMPRESSIONS **1 BREATH**

**If a child is not breathing
and has no pulse, give cycles
of 5 compressions and
1 breath.**

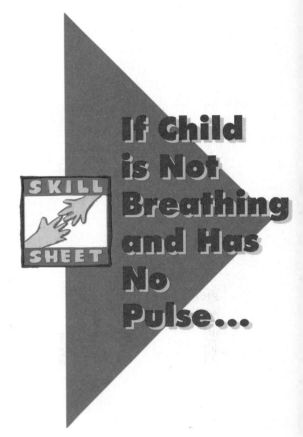

If Child is Not Breathing and Has No Pulse...

SKILL SHEET

hand on the breastbone in the middle of the child's chest and then push down and let up five times. Each compression should be about 1½ inches deep. These 5 compressions should take about 3 seconds. Count, "one, two, three, . . ." to help you maintain an even and regular rhythm.

After giving 5 compressions, you must get oxygen into the child's lungs. With the head tilted back, lift the chin, and give 1 slow breath (for about 1½ seconds) until the chest rises. Continue this cycle of 5 compressions and 1 breath. Do about 12 cycles of CPR (about one minute). Then recheck pulse and breathing. If you can't feel the pulse, continue CPR until help arrives. Recheck every few minutes for pulse and breathing.

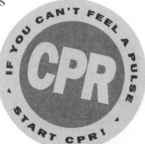

IF YOU CAN'T FEEL A PULSE **CPR** START CPR!

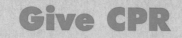

Give CPR

The emergency number has been called. If, when you check, the person is not breathing and has no pulse...

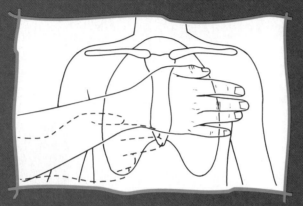

STEP 1

Find hand position on about the center of the breastbone.

STEP 2

Position shoulders over hands. Compress chest 5 times.

STEP 3

Give 1 slow breath.

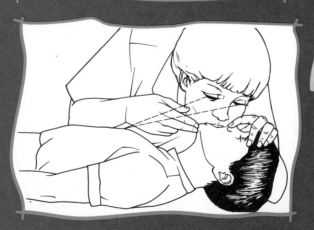

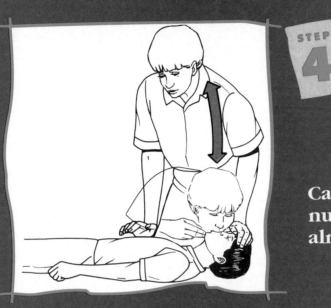

STEP 4

Repeat cycles of 5 compressions and 1 breath for about 1 minute (about 12 cycles).

Call the local emergency number if you have not already done so. Then...

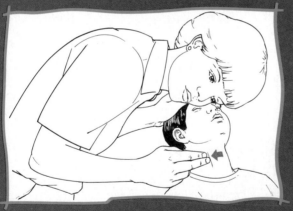

STEP 5

Recheck pulse and breathing for about 5 seconds.

If there is still no pulse ...

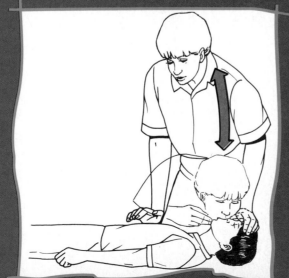

STEP 6

Continue sets of 5 compressions and 1 breath. Recheck pulse and breathing every few minutes.

Caring for *Infants* With Breathing Emergencies

It was noted in the previous article that the care for infants (birth to 1 year) and children with breathing and cardiac emergencies is similar. Care differs in a few areas because infants and children vary in size. In general the skills presented here should be used for an infant under 1 year of age. If you are uncertain of the infant's age, use your own judgment. If an infant is too long or too heavy for you to support him or her on your arm and hand, especially if the infant is choking, use the technique for a child.

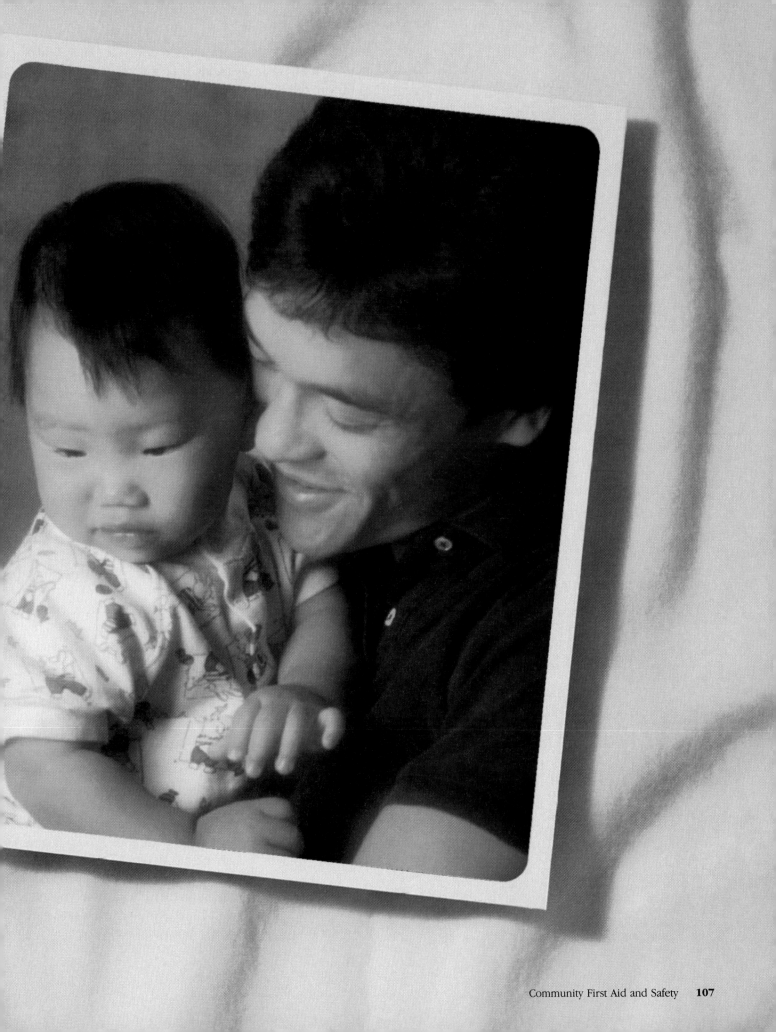

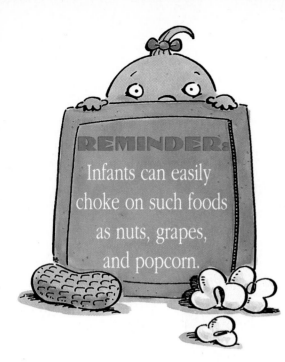

REMINDER:
Infants can easily choke on such foods as nuts, grapes, and popcorn.

If an Infant Is Choking

Choking is a major cause of death and injury in infants. One reason is that infants learn about their world by putting objects in their mouths. Small objects, such as pebbles, coins, beads, and parts of toys, are dangerous if an infant puts them in the mouth. Infants also often choke because it takes a long time to develop their eating skills. Infants can easily choke on some foods that an adult can eat, such as nuts, grapes, or popcorn.

To prevent choking, never let an infant eat alone. Never prop up a bottle for an infant to drink alone.

Always stay with an infant during meals or snacks. Cut food into small pieces. Do not give an infant foods, such as nuts, that could lodge in the airway. If you suspect that an infant has an object in his or her mouth, check with your fingers and remove it. Regularly check floors, rugs, and other places for pins, coins, and other small objects that an infant might pick up and put in his or her mouth.

Like a child who is choking, a choking infant can quickly stop breathing, lose consciousness, and die. If the infant is coughing forcefully, allow the infant to continue to cough. Watch the infant carefully. If the infant does not stop coughing in a few minutes or if the infant coughs weakly, makes a high-pitched sound while coughing, or cannot cry, cough, or breathe, have someone call the local emergency number for help. To clear a blocked airway, you will need to give back blows and chest thrusts.

To do this, position the infant facedown on your arm, with your hand supporting the infant's head. With your other hand, strike the infant between the shoulder blades 5 times. Turn the infant over, place two or three fingers in the center of the breastbone, and give 5 chest thrusts. Each thrust should be about 1 inch deep. Turn the infant facedown again and repeat back blows, followed by chest thrusts.

Stop as soon as the object is coughed up or the infant starts to breathe or cough. Watch the infant and make sure that he or she is breathing freely again. Call the local emergency number if you have not already done so. The infant should be taken to the hospital emergency department to be checked by a doctor. Do this even if the infant seems to be breathing well.

To clear a blocked airway, you will need to repeat a series of 5 back blows and 5 chest thrusts.

BACK 5 BLOWS   CHEST 5 THRUSTS

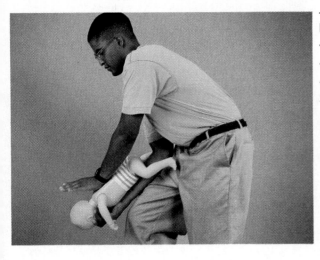

Position the infant facedown on your forearm so that the head is lower than the chest. Give 5 back blows between the shoulder blades (*top*). Turn the infant onto his or her back (*middle*). Give 5 chest thrusts in the center of the breastbone (*bottom*).

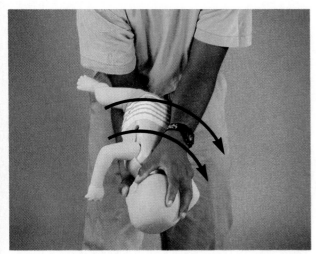

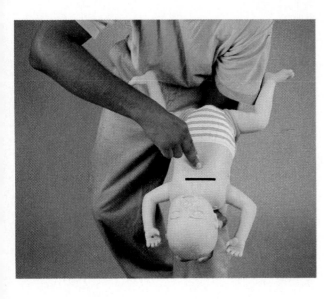

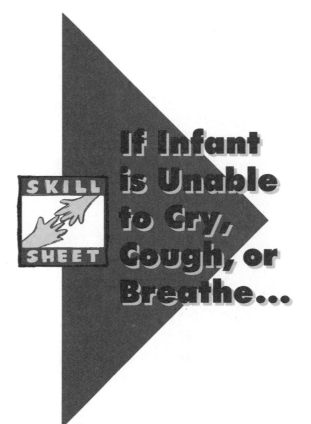

SKILL SHEET

If Infant is Unable to Cry, Cough, or Breathe...

Give Back Blows and Chest Thrusts

If, when you check, the infant is unable to cough, cry, or breathe. . .

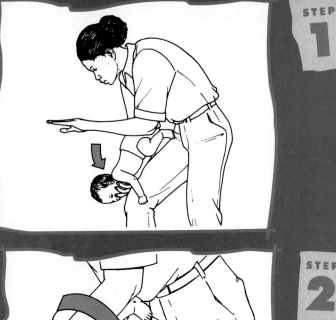

STEP 1

With infant facedown on forearm, give 5 back blows with heel of hand between infant's shoulder blades.

STEP 2

Position infant faceup on forearm.

STEP 3

Give 5 chest thrusts on about the center of the breastbone.

Repeat back blows and chest thrusts until object is coughed up, infant begins to breathe on own, or infant becomes unconscious.

An infant who is not breathing needs rescue breathing. Give 1 breath about every 3 seconds.

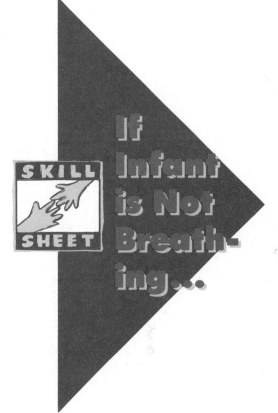

SKILL SHEET

If Infant is Not Breathing...

If an Infant Is Not Breathing

When an infant stops breathing, his or her body can function for only a few minutes without oxygen before body systems begin to fail. Like a child, an infant who is not breathing but has a pulse needs rescue breathing immediately. Rescue breathing provides the oxygen the infant needs to survive. You discover whether you need to give rescue breathing when you check the infant's breathing and pulse. You do not need to tip an infant's head back very far to open the airway. You will know the airway is open if you can see the infant's chest rise and fall as you give breaths.

Because an infant's mouth is so small, you should seal your mouth over the infant's mouth and nose instead of just over the mouth as you would for a child. Breathe slowly into the infant only until you see the chest rise. Each breath should last about 1½ seconds. Pause in between breaths to let the air flow back out. Watch the chest rise each time you breathe in to be sure that your breaths are actually going in. Give 1 breath about every 3 seconds. A good way to time the breaths is to count "one one-thousand," take a breath yourself on "two one-thousand," and breathe into the infant on "three one-thousand." Remember to breathe slowly and gently. Breathing too hard or too fast can force air into the infant's stomach.

After 1 minute of rescue breathing (about 20 breaths), recheck the infant's pulse. If the infant still has a pulse but is not breathing, continue rescue breathing. Check the pulse every minute. Continue rescue breathing until help arrives.

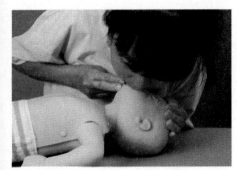

To give rescue breaths to an infant, seal your mouth over the infant's mouth and nose.

Give Rescue Breathing

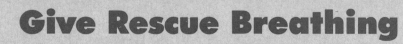

The emergency number has been called. If, when you check, the infant is not breathing. . .

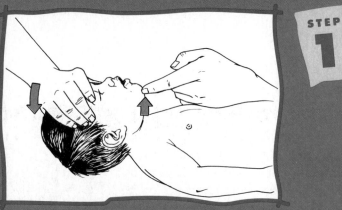

STEP 1

Keep head tilted back.

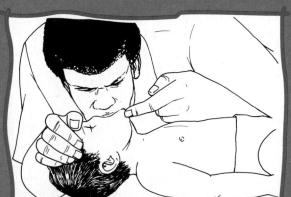

STEP 2

Seal your lips tightly around infant's mouth and nose.

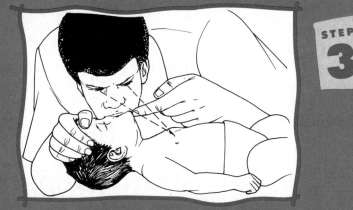

STEP 3

Give 2 slow breaths. Breathe into infant until chest gently rises.

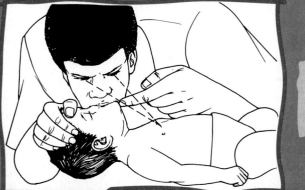

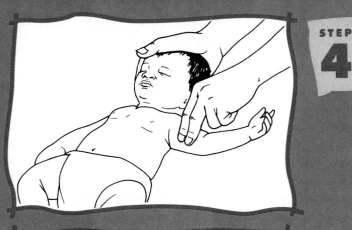

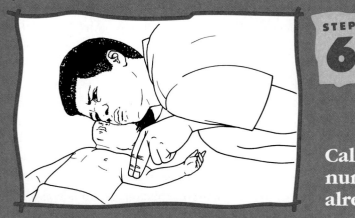

STEP 4 Check for a pulse.

If pulse is present but infant is still not breathing ...

STEP 5 Give 1 slow breath about every 3 seconds. Do this for about 1 minute (20 breaths).

STEP 6 Recheck pulse and breathing.

Call the local emergency number if you have not already done so. Then, continue rescue breathing as long as pulse is present but infant is not breathing. Recheck pulse and breathing about every minute.

SIDS

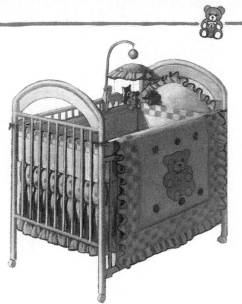

"**F**or the first few months, I would lie awake in bed at night and wonder if she was still breathing. I mean you just never know. I couldn't get to sleep until I checked on her at least once." This is how one mother described her first experience with parenting.

Sudden Infant Death Syndrome (SIDS) is the sudden, unexpected, and unexplained death of apparently healthy babies. It is the major cause of death for infants between the ages of 1 month and 1 year. In the United States, SIDS, sometimes called crib death, is responsible for the death of about 7,000 infants each year.

Because it cannot be predicted or prevented, SIDS causes many new parents to feel anxious. With no warning signs or symptoms, a sleeping infant can stop breathing and never wake again. Parents and other family members of SIDS victims often have trouble dealing with this traumatic event. Along with the stress of mourning their loss, they endure tremendous feelings of guilt, believing that they should have been able to prevent the child's death.

Some basic facts about SIDS:

- Ninety percent of SIDS deaths occur while the infant is asleep.
- SIDS deaths can occur between the ages of 2 weeks and 18 months. Ninety five percent of deaths occur between 2 and 4 months of age.
- The majority of SIDS deaths occur in fall and winter.
- Between 30 and 50 percent of SIDS victims have minor respiratory or gastrointestinal infections at the time of death.
- SIDS occurs slightly more often in boys than in girls.

For more information, call the National SIDS Resource Center at (703) 821-8955, ext. 249 or 474.

Researchers are working to find the cause(s) of SIDS. At this time, several risk factors—characteristics that occur more often in SIDS victims than in normal babies—have been discovered. Yet these risk factors are not causes and cannot be used to predict which infants will die. For example, 95 percent of SIDS deaths occur in infants between 2 and 4 months of age, so being in this age group is a risk factor. Other risk factors for SIDS include smoking during pregnancy, first pregnancy under 20 years of age, several children already born to the mother, a baby with a low birthweight, and a baby with a low growth rate during the mother's pregnancy.

The best prevention for SIDS, as well as many other infant diseases, is for pregnant women to practice healthy behaviors while pregnant. They should get proper prenatal care, eat a balanced diet, not smoke or drink alcoholic drinks, and get adequate rest and exercise.

REFERENCES

National SIDS Resource Center (formerly National SIDS Clearinghouse). *Fact Sheet: SIDS Information for the EMT.* McLean, VA, 1990.

Department of Health and Human Services, Public Health Service, Health Resources and Services Administration, Maternal and Child Health Bureau. *Information Exchange: Newsletter of the National SIDS Clearinghouse.* IE32, July 1991.

If Air Won't Go In

If the infant's chest doesn't rise when you give breaths, the airway is probably blocked. It may be blocked by the infant's tongue or an object. If the infant was left alone with a bottle to drink, fluids may be blocking the airway.

You must clear the blockage immediately. First, retilt the infant's head and lift the chin. Try to give breaths again. If the breaths still don't go in, you must assume there is something blocking the airway and try to remove it. Use the same combination of back blows and chest thrusts that you used for the conscious infant.

Give 5 back blows between the shoulder blades while you hold the infant facedown on your forearm.

Then give 5 chest thrusts on the lower part of the breastbone while the infant is supported on your arm. Next, look in the infant's mouth for the object. If you can see it, remove it with your finger. Then give 2 breaths to try to get oxygen into the infant's lungs. Continue the back blows, chest thrusts, checks for object, and breaths until the infant coughs the object up or begins to breathe or cough.

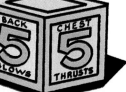

If you are unable to breathe into an infant, the airway is probably blocked. Give 5 back blows and 5 chest thrusts.

If Air Does Not Go In...

SKILL SHEET

Give Back Blows and Chest Thrusts

The emergency number has been called. If, when you check, the infant is not breathing and your breaths do not go in...

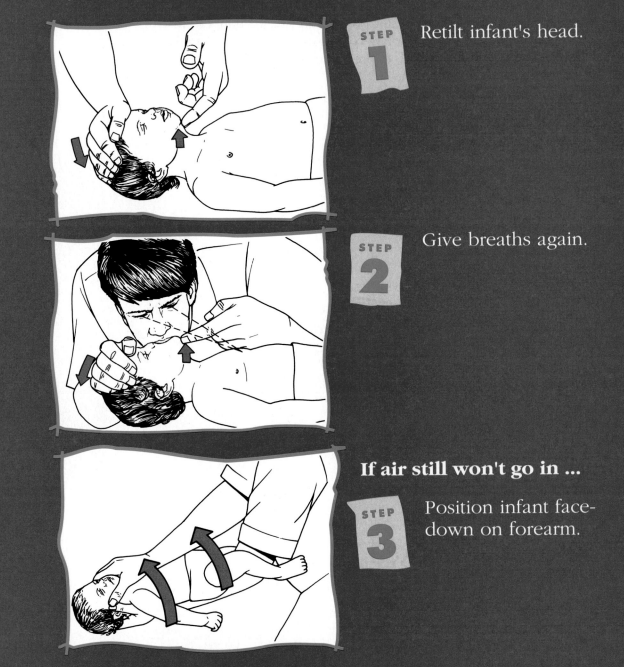

STEP 1 Retilt infant's head.

STEP 2 Give breaths again.

If air still won't go in ...

STEP 3 Position infant face-down on forearm.

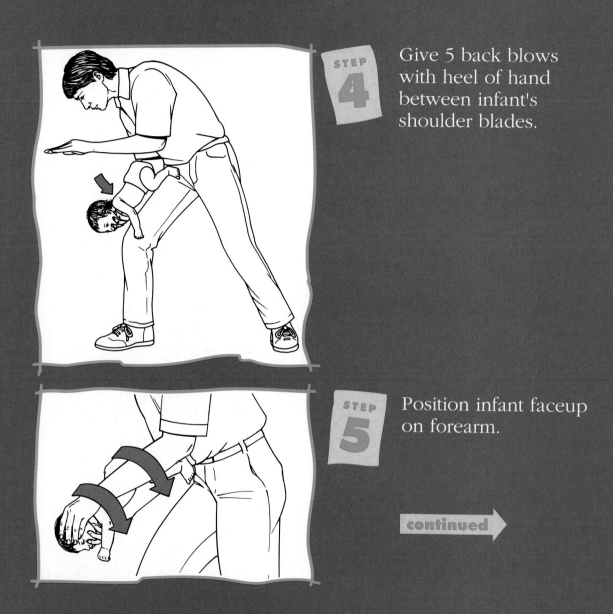

STEP 4

Give 5 back blows with heel of hand between infant's shoulder blades.

STEP 5

Position infant faceup on forearm.

continued →

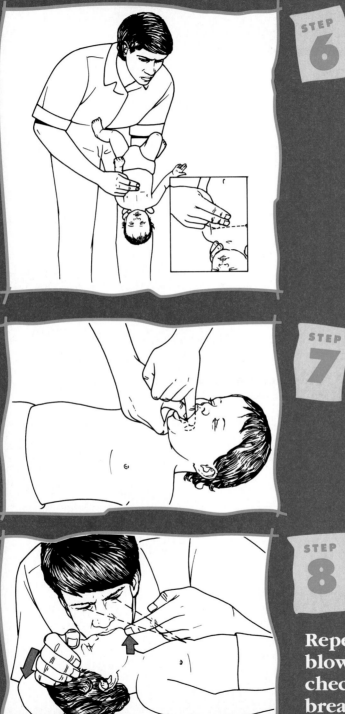

STEP 6

Give 5 chest thrusts on about the center of the breastbone.

STEP 7

Lift jaw and tongue and check for object. If object is seen, sweep it out with finger.

STEP 8

Tilt head back and give breaths again.

Repeat breaths, back blows, chest thrusts, and checks for object until breaths go in.

Call the local emergency number after giving care for 1 minute if you have not already done so.

If an Infant Does Not Have a Pulse

An infant who is not breathing and does not have a pulse needs CPR. Feel for an infant's pulse on the inside of the upper arm, between the infant's elbow and shoulder. Start CPR if you can't feel the pulse after checking for about 5 seconds.

To give CPR, place the infant on his or her back on a hard surface, such as the floor or a table. If you have to move the infant to the telephone so you can call for help, the hard surface can be your hand or forearm, with your palm supporting the infant's back. Place two fingers on the breastbone just below an imaginary line between the nipples and give 5 compressions. These should take about 3 seconds. Count "one, two, three, four, five, . . ." to help keep a regular and even rhythm.

After giving 5 compressions, give 1 slow breath (about 1½ seconds). Then begin compressions again. Do 12 cycles of 5 compressions and 1 breath (about 1 minute). Then recheck the pulse. If you can't feel the pulse, continue with cycles of 5 compressions and 1 breath until help arrives. Check every few minutes for pulse and breathing.

Ask someone to call the local emergency number as soon as you find out that the infant is unconscious. If you are alone, give CPR for about 1 minute, then make the call yourself. If you can, carry the infant to the telephone so that you can continue giving CPR.

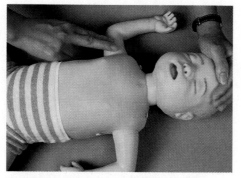

Feel for an infant's pulse on the inside of the upper arm, between the infant's elbow and shoulder.

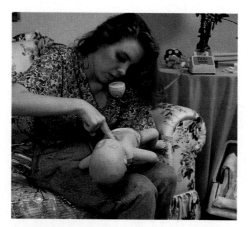

The hard surface of your hand or forearm can be used to support an infant during CPR if you have to move to a phone.

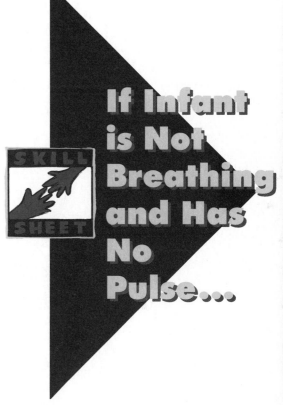

If Infant is Not Breathing and Has No Pulse...

SKILL SHEET

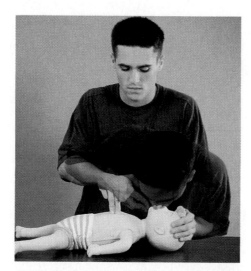

An infant who is not breathing and does not have a pulse needs CPR. Alternate giving 5 chest compressions and 1 breath.

Give CPR

The emergency number has been called. If, when you check, the infant is not breathing and has no pulse...

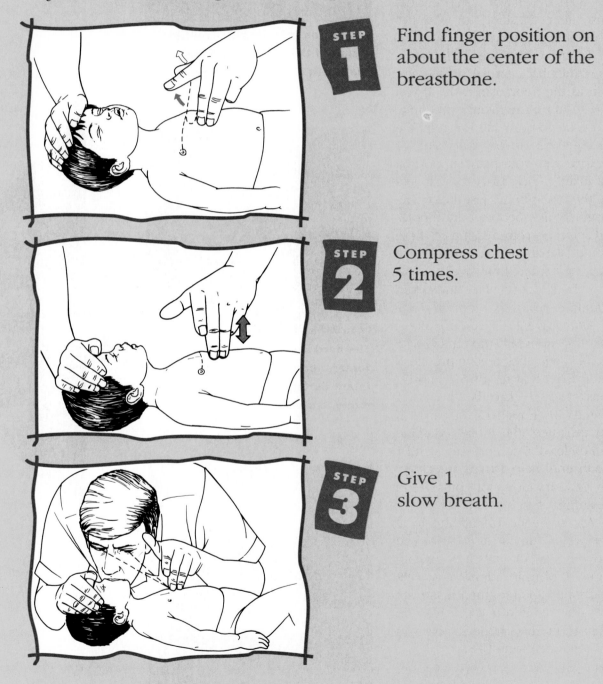

STEP 1
Find finger position on about the center of the breastbone.

STEP 2
Compress chest 5 times.

STEP 3
Give 1 slow breath.

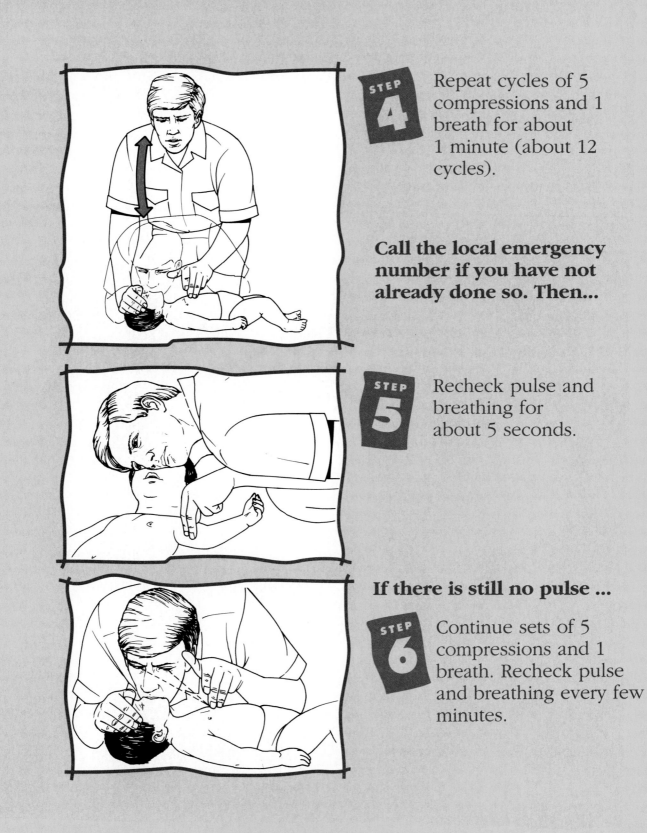

STEP 4

Repeat cycles of 5 compressions and 1 breath for about 1 minute (about 12 cycles).

Call the local emergency number if you have not already done so. Then...

STEP 5

Recheck pulse and breathing for about 5 seconds.

If there is still no pulse ...

STEP 6

Continue sets of 5 compressions and 1 breath. Recheck pulse and breathing every few minutes.

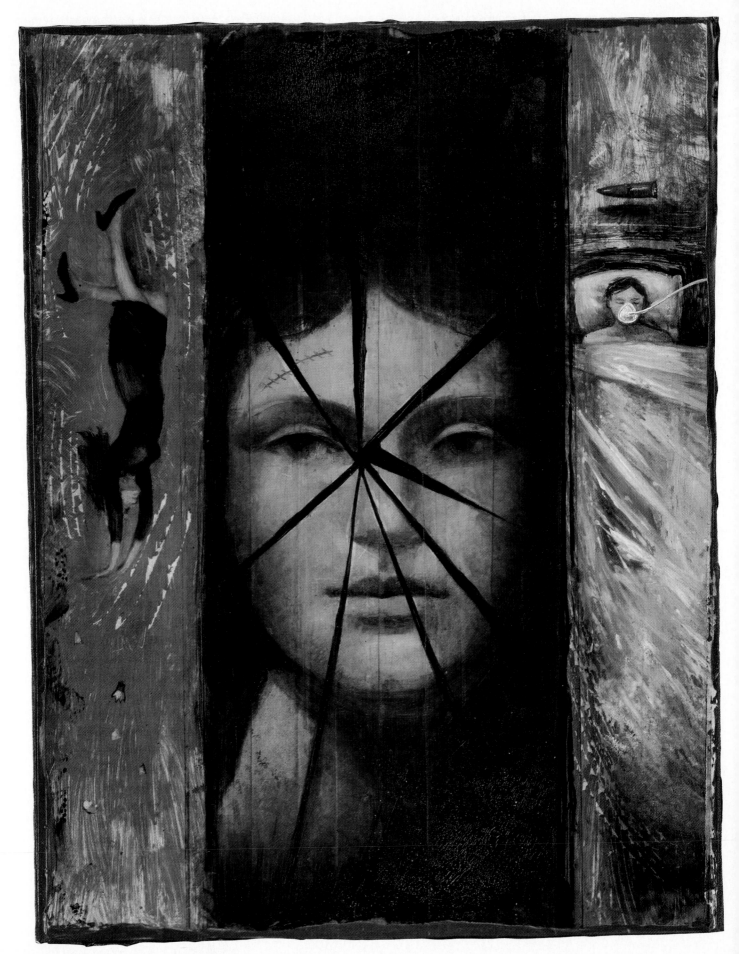

The wail of sirens breaks the sleepy afternoon stillness. A police car suddenly pulls to a stop on the shady street and an officer goes into a house. An ambulance drives up and two paramedics dart into the house. Another ambulance quickly arrives and still others head toward the house. For a few moments all is quiet. Suddenly several people emerge from the house carrying a stretcher. On it is a body—not very large. Paramedics cluster around the body, frantically trying to save the child's life. They slide the stretcher into the ambulance. A distraught woman runs after them. She turns to the police officer next to her. "I don't know where he found the gun," she chokes. "My husband keeps it in his desk. It couldn't have been loaded."

INJURIES

Injury is one of our nation's most important health problems. Most of us will have a significant injury at some time in our lives. In the few minutes it takes you to read this information, two people will be killed and 170 will suffer disabling injuries. Besides the cost in grief and pain, these injuries will cost $2,700,000 in lost income, medical expenses, property damage, insurance, and other costs.

Causes of Injury

Injuries that damage, disable, and kill are caused by different types of force. For example, a blow to the chest can break ribs. Another example is the force of a bullet that

M ost of us will have a significant injury at some time in our lives.

travels through skin and muscle, striking a blood vessel and causing serious bleeding within the body.

Sometimes, a force causes an injury to an area in the body away from the area where it strikes. This happens, for example, when you fall and hit the floor with an outstretched hand and the force of the impact travels up your arm, injuring your shoulder.

Moving your body in certain ways also causes injuries. Even movements as simple as stepping off a curb or turning to reach for an out-of-the-way object can cause injury. Suddenly contracting, or tightening, a muscle or group of muscles can also cause injury. These types of muscle injuries commonly

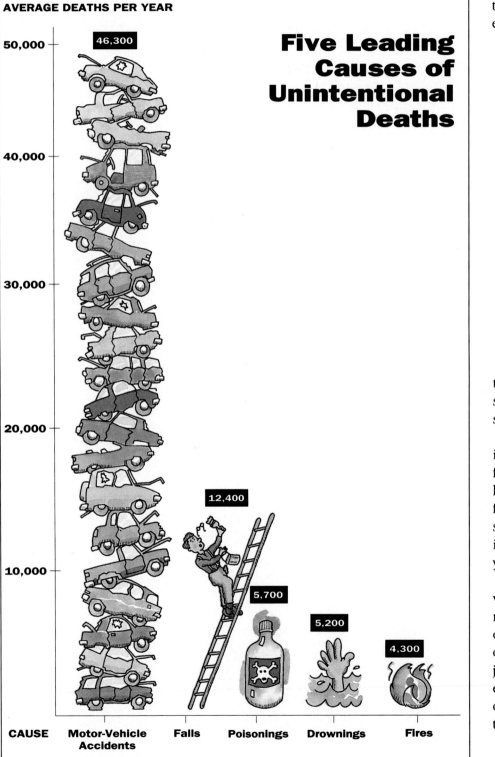

AVERAGE DEATHS PER YEAR

Five Leading Causes of Unintentional Deaths

50,000 — 46,300

40,000 —

30,000 —

20,000 —

12,400

10,000 — 5,700

5,200

4,300

CAUSE Motor-Vehicle Accidents   Falls   Poisonings   Drownings   Fires

National Safety Council. *Accident Facts,* 1991.

happen in sports activities, some-times as a result of not warming up enough.

You can also be injured by the energy from heat, chemicals, radia-tion, and electricity, which all cause burns. Thousands die each year from fires and burns. They are the fifth leading cause of unintentional death. Most of these fatal injuries happen at home. Fires cause 66 percent of all deaths from burns. Hot liquids cause 27 percent, and electricity causes only 1 percent. The most common causes of nonfa-tal burns are scalds from hot liq-uids or foods and contact with hot surfaces. Over 1 million burn inju-ries a year require medical care. Over 90,000 people with burns stay in a hospital for an average of 12 days.

Reducing Your Risk of Injury

How does this information relate to you? What are your chances of in-

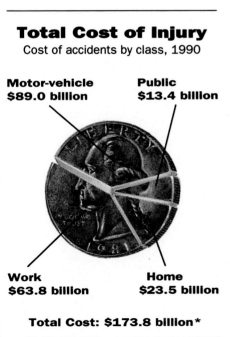

Total Cost of Injury
Cost of accidents by class, 1990

Motor-vehicle $89.0 billion

Public $13.4 billion

Work $63.8 billion

Home $23.5 billion

Total Cost: $173.8 billion*

*Duplication between motor-vehicle and work was $15.9 million.
National Safety Council. *Accident Facts,* 1991.

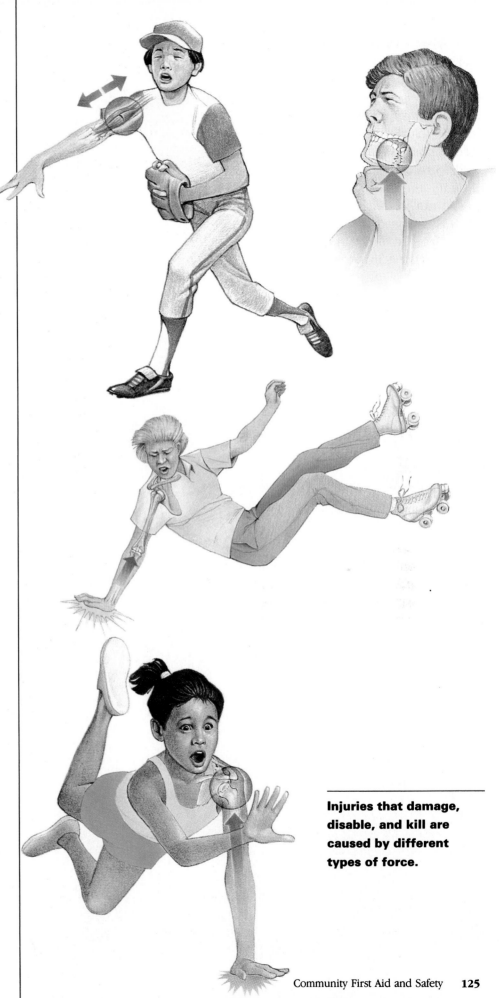

Injuries that damage, disable, and kill are caused by different types of force.

jury? What can you do to reduce your risk of injury?

People of certain ages are injured more often than others. Injury rates are higher for people under 45. Injuries resulting in death occur most often among people aged 15 to 24. Men are more likely to be injured than women.

Do not be misled by these figures. The reason the injury rate is higher for certain groups has more to do with the activities of the group than with the group itself. Your chances of an injury and the extent of

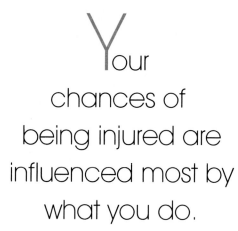

Your chances of being injured are influenced most by what you do.

that injury have more to do with what you do than with who you are.

Many people believe that injuries just happen. They believe that those who are injured are just unfortunate victims of circumstance, but this is not true. Overwhelming evidence exists that injuries, like disease, do not just happen. Rather, many injuries are predictable, preventable events resulting from the way people interact with the potential dangers in the environment. There are three general strategies for preventing injuries:
• Persuade people at risk to change their behavior.

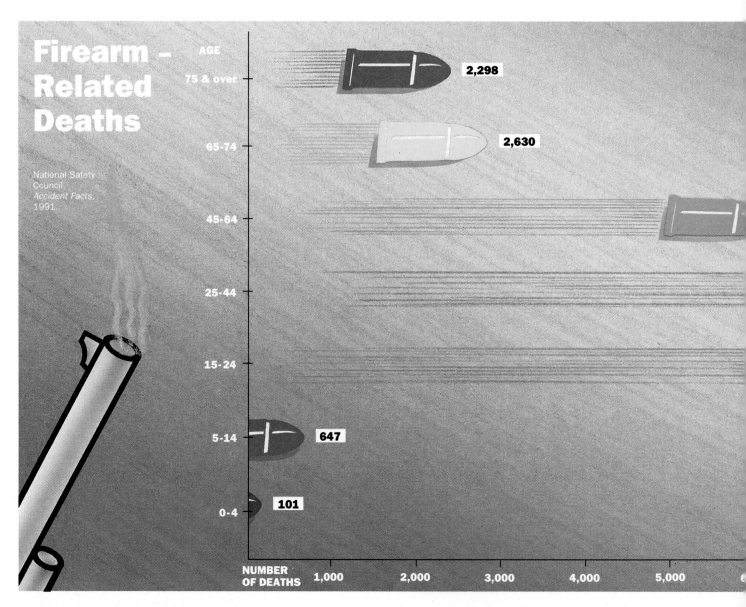

Firearm – Related Deaths

National Safety Council, *Accident Facts*, 1991.

AGE	
75 & over	2,298
65-74	2,630
45-64	
25-44	
15-24	
5-14	647
0-4	101

NUMBER OF DEATHS   1,000   2,000   3,000   4,000   5,000

- Require people at risk to change their behavior.
- Provide automatic protection products designed to reduce the risk of injury.

Although laws that require you to take safety measures, such as wearing safety belts, are moderately effective, the most successful injury-prevention strategy is the protection built into the product. Automatic protection, such as airbags in motor vehicles, does not allow people to make choices.

Typically, behaviors of mem-

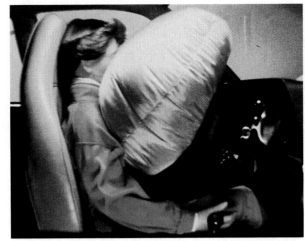

Insurance Institute for Highway Safety

Automatic protection, such as airbags in motor vehicles, does not allow people to make choices about safety.

Firearm deaths are rising at an alarming rate in the United States. Since 1953, deaths from firearms have more than doubled. Although accidental deaths have decreased, suicides have more than doubled and homicides have more than tripled.

In 1988, over 80% of firearm deaths were in males. Although suicide totals are highest for those aged 25 to 44, the death rate per 100,000 population is highest for 75 years and over. For homicides, total deaths are highest for the 25 to 44 year age group, but death rates are highest for those aged 15 to 24.

National Safety Council. *Accident Facts*, 1991.

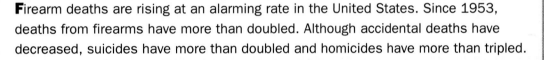

14,207

7,805

| 7,000 | 8,000 | 9,000 | 10,000 | 11,000 | 12,000 | 13,000 | 14,000 | 15,000 |

WATCH YOUR BAC!

What's *your* BAC? Not a question you would usually be able to answer, but if you are suspected of driving drunk, the police will find the answer by taking a blood, breath, or urine sample and analyzing it. BAC stands for blood alcohol concentration. The test result is expressed as a blood alcohol concentration percentage.

In the United States, each state has set a legal limit for BAC. States punish those who choose to drive drunk with fines, loss of license, or jail. In most states a driver with a BAC of 0.10 percent or more is considered to be driving while intoxicated (DWI). For a 140-pound person, reaching this blood alcohol level takes about three drinks in 1 hour. One drink equals 12 oz. of beer, 5 oz. of wine, or 1½ oz. of hard liquor.

Although BAC limits have been established for lawful driving, a lower BAC can still impair the physical and mental abilities you need to drive safely. Your judgment, coordination, and reaction times are all dulled by alcohol. Researchers estimate that the risk of being involved in a fatal crash may be at least eight times higher for a drunk driver than for a sober one.

Motor vehicle crashes are a major cause of death from injury in the United States. In 1989, 47,575 people died in traffic crashes.[1] About one half of these deaths were alcohol related.[2] Traffic deaths and crashes involving alcohol occur most often to people who are 18 to 24 years of age.[3] Young people are often less used to alcohol and take more risk.

Think before you drink.

• Set a limit, such as one drink per hour, and stick to it.

NUMBER OF DRINKS

BODY WEIGHT	1	2	3	4	5
100	.04	.09	.15	.20	.25
120	.03	.08	.12	.16	.21
140	.02	.06	.10	.14	.18
160	.02	.05	.09	.12	.15
180	.02	.05	.08	.10	.13
200	.01	.04	.07	.09	.12

The amount of alcohol in mixed drinks varies considerably, depending on the recipe and type of liquor used.

Figures are rounded to nearest .01. BACs shown are approximate, since they can be affected by factors other than weight.

0 to .04
Not legally under the influence. Impairment possible.

.05 to .09
State laws vary. Mental and physical impairment noticeable.

.10 and above
Presumed intoxicated in all 50 states.

National Clearinghouse for Alcohol Information

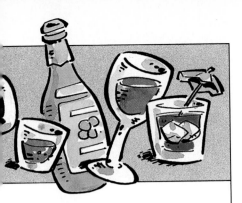

- Eat before and as you drink to slow the absorption of alcohol into your system.

- Switch to nonalcoholic beverages like juice or soda when you've reached your limit.

- Never drink and drive — choose a driver who agrees not to drink, take public transportation, or stay overnight.

- Exercise your right to say "no thanks" to the first drink or to any other drink.

- Be honest with yourself—realize that even one drink can increase your risk of injuring yourself or someone else.

For more information about how to prevent alcohol-related deaths and injuries, contact your local chapters of Mothers Against Drunk Driving (MADD) and Students Against Drunk Driving (SADD).

REFERENCES

1. Centers for Disease Control. *Monthly Vital Statistics Report*, 40 (8), Supplement 2. January 1992.

2. National Highway Traffic Safety Administration. *Alcohol Involvement in Fatal Traffic Crashes, 1989*. February 1991.

3. National Safety Council. *Accident Facts*, 1991.

SAFETY YES! INJURY NO!

Reducing Your Risk of Injury

Take measures that can decrease your risk of injury and the risk to others.

Think safety—be alert and avoid potentially harmful conditions or activities that increase your injury risk.

Take precautions, such as wearing appropriate protective devices— helmets, padding, and eyewear— and buckle up when driving or riding in motor vehicles.

Let your state and congressional representatives know that you support legislation that ensures a safer environment for us all.

bers of high-risk groups tend to be the hardest to influence. For example, despite the overwhelming number of traffic deaths in the 15-to-19 age group, teenagers are less likely than adults to wear seat belts.

Many people view laws that require certain behaviors as an infringement of their rights—even though the laws are intended to protect them from injury. Product designs are also difficult to influence because many manufacturers are reluctant to spend the money for design changes. For instance, the evidence in favor of safety belts was available many years ago. However, it took over 20 years of fighting to get a federal regulation requiring automobile manufacturers to install automatic restraints by 1990. The American Trauma Society

If existing information about prevention were applied, the injury rate could be reduced by 50 percent.

contends that, if all of the existing information about prevention were applied, the injury rate could be reduced by 50 percent.

Although there are some injury factors that you can do little about, there are others that you directly control. For example, drinking alcohol is a primary cause of many injuries and deaths, especially from motor vehicle accidents. Many people who die from falls, drowning, fires, and suicides have more than the legal limit of alcohol in their blood. Alcohol is also a factor in about 20 percent of those injured at home, 16 percent of those injured on the job, and 56 percent of those injured in fights and assaults. *You* can control where, when, and how much you drink.

Taking precautions also helps cut down on injuries. This is shown by the reduced numbers of deaths from motor vehicle crashes since people began wearing safety belts. Whether or not to wear a safety belt is *your* decision.

Injuries do not just happen. For the most part, they are predictable and preventable. If you haven't already done so, answer the Injury Prevention IQ Quiz on page 131. This questionnaire will help heighten your awareness of conditions or situations around you that may lead to injury. It may help you reduce your risk of injury, as well as risk to others.

Each year in the United States, thousands of people will die, millions will be injured, and over 100 billion dollars will be spent, all needlessly. The cause... many injuries that could have been prevented.

REFERENCES

National Safety Council. *Accident Facts*, 1991.

U.S. Department of Health and Human Services, Public Health Service. *Healthy People 2000, National Health Promotion and Disease Prevention Objectives.* Washington, D.C., 1990.

Mark "yes" or "no" to the following questions:

[Y] [N] Do you wear a safety belt when driving or riding in a motor vehicle?

[Y] [N] Do you refrain from operating motor vehicles after drinking alcoholic beverages?

[Y] [N] If you own a gun, do you keep it unloaded and locked in a safe place?

[Y] [N] Do the stairs where you live have hand rails?

[Y] [N] Do you use a stepladder or sturdy stool to reach high, out-of-reach objects?

[Y] [N] Do you have adequate lighting in halls and stairways?

[Y] [N] Do you use good lifting technique when lifting objects?

[Y] [N] Do you wear a helmet when riding a bicycle, motorcycle, or skateboard?

[Y] [N] Do you wear a lifejacket when participating in activities on or near the water?

[Y] [N] Do you wear safety protection (i.e., goggles and hearing protection) and follow equipment safety recommendations when operating power tools?

If you answered "no" to any of these questions, consider that in the United States—

- Half of all deaths from unintentional injuries are a result of motor vehicle crashes.

- Alcohol use is a factor in about half of all motor vehicle fatalities.

- The number of firearm deaths has doubled since 1953. About 15 percent of all firearm-related deaths are unintentional, often resulting from improper handling, accessibility to children, and lack of safety mechanisms.

- Falls account for the largest number of preventable injuries for persons over 75 years of age.

- Injuries to the back make up 22 percent of all disabling injuries in the workplace.

- Almost 30 percent of all motor vehicle fatalities are related to bicycle, pedestrian, and motorcycle casualties. Increasing helmet usage should reduce the number of fatalities.

- In 1988, there were about 5,000 deaths resulting from drowning. Over half of all drowning victims are between the ages of 15 and 44.

- Injuries to the eyes, hands, or fingers make up 22 percent of all disabling injuries in the workplace.

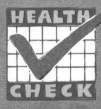

HEALTH CHECK

INJURY PREVENTION

IQ QUIZ

CUTS, SCRAPES, & BRUISES

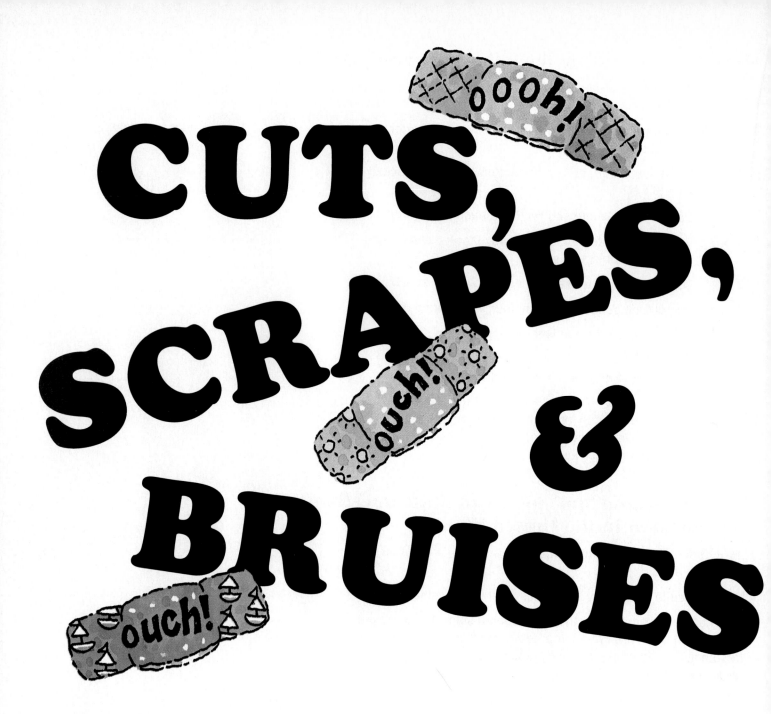

A baby falls and bruises his arm while learning to walk. A toddler scrapes her knee while learning to run. A child needs stitches in his chin after he falls off the monkey bars on the playground. A teenager gets a black eye in a fist fight. A college student suffers a sunburn during a weekend at the beach. An adult cuts his hand while working in a woodshop. What do all these injuries have in common? They are all soft tissue injuries.

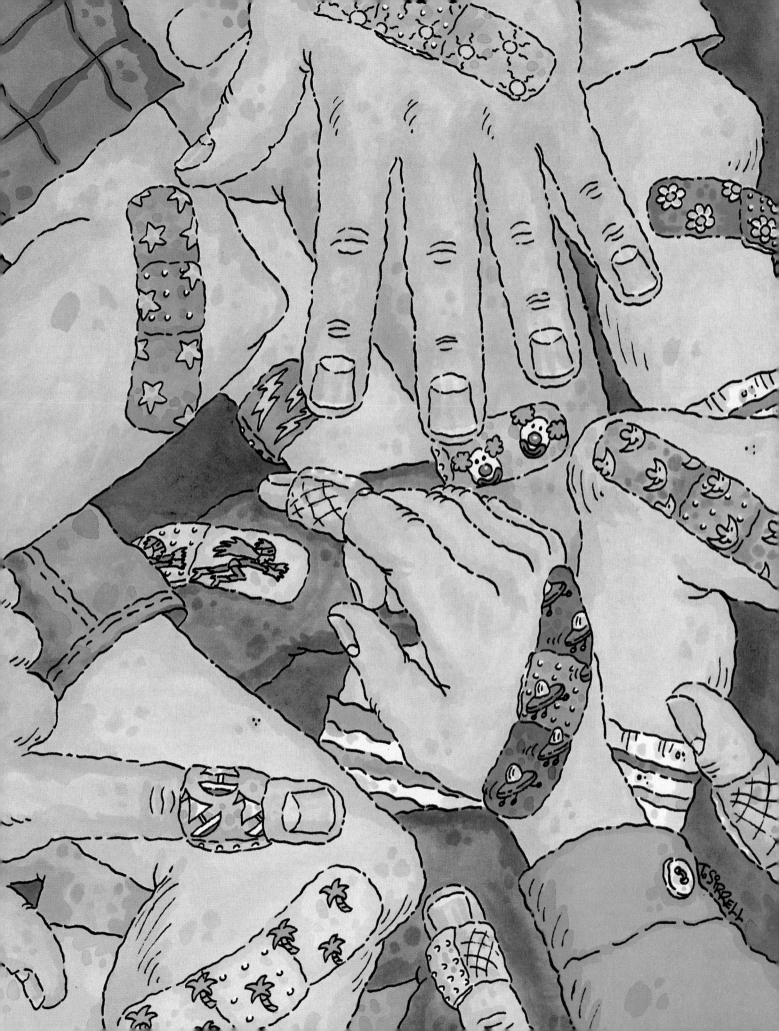

Soft tissues are the layers of skin and the fat and muscle beneath the skin. Anytime the soft tissues are damaged or torn, the body is threatened. Injuries may damage the soft tissues at or near the skin's surface or deep in the body. Severe bleeding can occur at the skin's surface and under it, where it is harder to detect. Germs can get into the body through a scrape, cut, or puncture and cause infection.

Burns are a special kind of soft tissue injury. Like other types of soft tissue injury, burns can damage only the top layer of skin or the skin and the layers of fat, muscle, and bone beneath.

An injury to the soft tissues is commonly called a wound. A wound is "closed" when the damage to the soft tissues is under the skin's surface, like a bruise. A bruise indicates bleeding under the skin. A wound is "open" when the skin's surface is broken. Scrapes, cuts, and punctures are open wounds. Avulsions are open wounds in which a piece of skin, soft tissue, or even part of the body,

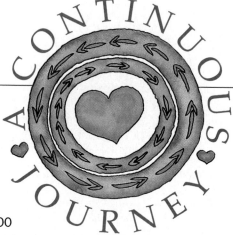

A CONTINUOUS JOURNEY

There are about 60,000 miles of blood vessels in your body. These vessels act as a road map, directing blood to all parts of the body. As long as your heart beats, blood will flow through a continuous circuit of blood vessels known as arteries, veins, and capillaries.

These blood vessels vary in diameter. The larger the vessel, the more blood that can flow through it. During rest, the heart pumps about 5 liters of blood per minute through the blood vessels. During exercise, the blood vessels handle as much as six times this amount. This requires the blood vessels to be able to expand.

Arteries are large blood vessels that carry blood from the heart to all parts of the body. Because the blood in the arteries is closer to the pumping action of the heart, blood in the arteries travels faster and under greater pressure than blood in capillaries and veins. Blood flow in the arteries pulses with the heartbeat. Therefore bleeding from the arteries is very fast and heavy. Arterial blood is usually bright red and because it is under pressure, it spurts from the wound. This is one easily recognizable signal of severe bleeding.

Veins return blood from the body to the heart. Bleeding from the veins is slower, steadier, and easier to control than arterial bleeding. Veins are damaged more often because they are closer to the skin's surface. Venous blood is dark red.

Capillaries are tiny blood vessels near the skin. They transfer oxygen and other nutrients to the body's cells. Bleeding from capillaries is usually slow and clots easily. The blood isn't as bright a red as blood from the arteries. Bleeding from scrapes and shallow cuts is from capillaries.

such as a finger, is torn loose or is torn off entirely.

Bleeding occurs when a blood vessel is torn. With any open wound, bleeding can be severe enough to be life-threatening. With

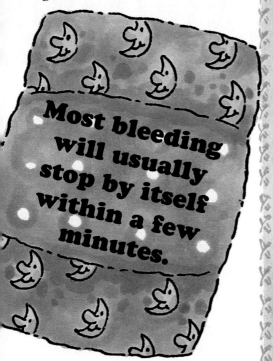

Most bleeding will usually stop by itself within a few minutes.

an open wound, the blood comes through a tear in the skin. Fortunately, most of the bleeding you will encounter will not be serious. It usually stops by itself within a few minutes. The blood at the wound clots and stops flowing. Sometimes, however, the damaged blood vessel is too large or the pressure in the blood vessel is too great for the blood to clot. Then bleeding can be life-threatening.

Scrapes are a common kind of open wound. They usually don't bleed very much. What bleeding they do cause comes from capillaries, the tiny blood vessels. Because dirt and germs are frequently rubbed into a wound when a scrape occurs, it is important to clean scrapes thoroughly to prevent infection.

Punctures are usually caused by a pointed object, such as a nail, piercing the skin. If the object remains in the wound, it is called an

A Stitch in Time

It can be difficult to judge when a wound should receive stitches from a doctor. One rule of thumb is that stitches are needed when edges of skin do not fall together or when any wound is over an inch long. Stitches speed the healing process, lessen the chances of infection, and improve the appearance of scars. They should be placed within the first few hours after the injury. The following major injuries often require stitches:

- Bleeding from an artery or uncontrolled bleeding
- Wounds that show muscle or bone, involve joints, gape widely, or involve hands or feet
- Large or deep puncture wounds
- Large or deeply embedded objects
- Human or animal bites
- Wounds that, if left unattended, could leave conspicuous scars, such as those on the face

If you are caring for a wound and think it may need stitches, it probably does. Once applied, stitches are easily cared for by dabbing them with hydrogen peroxide once or twice daily. If the wound gets red or swollen or if pus begins to form, notify your doctor.

Stitches in the face are often removed in less than a week. In joints, they are often removed after 2 weeks. Stitches on most other body parts require removal in 6 to 10 days. Some stitches dissolve naturally and do not require removal.

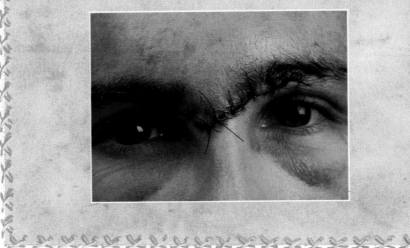

TYPES OF WOUNDS

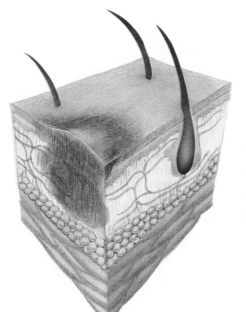

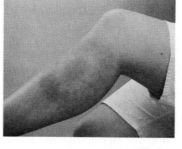

BRUISE
(Contusion; Charley Horse)

Damage to soft tissues and blood vessels causes bleeding under the skin. Tissues discolor and swell. At first, the area may only appear red. Over time, it may turn dark red or purple. A large or painful bruise may be a signal of severe damage to deep tissues.

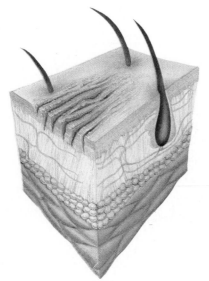

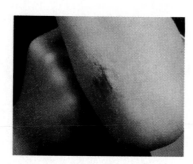

SCRAPE
(Abrasion; Road rash; Rug burn; Strawberry)

Most common type of wound. Caused by skin that has been rubbed or scraped away. Usually painful because scraping away of outer layer of skin exposes nerve endings. Dirt and other matter can easily become ground into the wound, making it especially important to clean it. Can easily become infected if not kept clean.

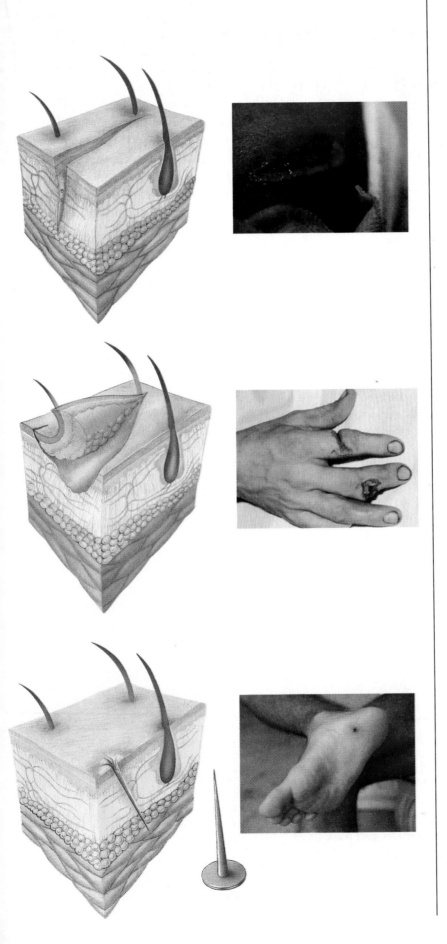

CUT
(Incision; Laceration)

A cut may have either jagged or smooth edges. Cuts are commonly caused by sharp-edged objects, such as knives, scissors, or broken glass. They can also result when a blow from a blunt object splits the skin. Deep cuts can damage nerves, large blood vessels, and other soft tissues. Cuts usually bleed freely. Deep cuts can bleed severely. A cut may not be painful if nerves are injured.

AVULSION

A cut in which a portion of skin or other soft tissue is partially or completely torn away. A partially avulsed piece of skin may remain but hangs like a flap. A violent force may completely tear away a body part, such as a finger. Because an avulsion often damages deeper tissues, bleeding is often significant. In contrast, when a body part is completely torn away, bleeding is easier to control because the tissues close around the vessels at the injury site.

PUNCTURE

A wound caused when a pointed object, such as a nail, piece of glass, or knife, pierces the skin. A gunshot wound is also a puncture wound. Because puncture wounds do not usually bleed a lot, they can easily become infected. Bleeding can be severe if the penetrating object damages major blood vessels or internal organs.
An object that remains embedded in the wound is called an impaled object. An object that passes completely through a body part will make two wounds—one at the entry point and one at the exit point.

Infection

When an injury breaks the skin, the best initial defense against infection is to clean the area. For minor wounds, wash the area with soap and water. Most soaps are effective in removing harmful bacteria. You do not need to wash wounds that require medical attention because they involve more extensive tissue damage or bleeding. It is more important to control the bleeding.

Because infected wounds can cause serious medical problems, it is important to maintain an up-to-date record of immunizations. These immunizations help your body fight infection. One of these immunizations prevents tetanus, a serious disease. The best way to prevent tetanus is to receive a booster shot every 5 to 10 years or whenever a wound is contaminated by a dirty object such as a rusty nail.

Sometimes, even the best care for a soft tissue injury is not enough to prevent infection. You will usually be able to recognize the early signals of infection. The area around the wound becomes swollen and red. The area may feel warm or throb with pain. Some wounds discharge pus. Serious infections may cause a person to develop a fever and feel ill. Red streaks may develop that progress from the wound in the direction of the heart.

If you see any of these signals of infection, care for the wound by keeping the area clean, soaking it in warm water, elevating the affected area, and applying an antibiotic ointment such as Neosporin. Change coverings over the wound daily. If fever or red streaks develop, the infection is getting worse. If the infection persists or worsens, seek medical help.

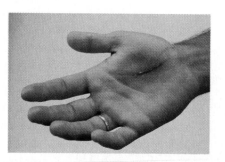

An infected wound may become swollen and may have a pus discharge.

impaled object. In most cases the object should not be removed. However, a splinter is an example of an impaled object that you can usually remove with tweezers if it is in the skin.

Punctures usually don't bleed very much unless a blood vessel has been injured. However, an object that goes into the soft tissues beneath the skin can carry germs deep into the body. These germs can cause infections, sometimes serious ones.

One severe infection that can result from a puncture or a deep cut is called tetanus. We all need to have the shot that protects us against tetanus and a booster shot every 5 to 10 years. Anyone whose skin is punctured or who is cut by an object that can carry infection, such as a rusty nail, or is bitten by an animal should check with his or her doctor to learn whether a booster shot is needed.

DRESSINGS AND BANDAGES

Open wounds need some type of covering to help control bleeding and prevent infection. These coverings are often called dressings and bandages. You can buy them at drugstores and many supermarkets.

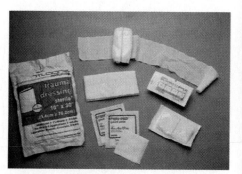

Dressings are pads placed directly on the wound. They come in various sizes. Some have surfaces that won't stick to a wound.

You should keep assorted sizes and shapes of dressings and bandages in your first aid kit.

Dressings are pads placed directly on the wound to soak up blood and help keep germs out. A dressing should be sterile (free from germs). Most dressings you buy are loosely woven to let air reach the wound. This helps the wound heal. Cotton gauze dressings 2 to 4 inches square are common. Some dressings have surfaces that won't stick to a wound.

A bandage is any material used to wrap or cover any part of the body. Bandages are often used to hold dressings in place, to apply pressure that helps control bleeding, and to help support an injured part of the body.

Bandages you can buy include small adhesive compresses such as Band-Aids, triangular bandages, roller bandages, and bandage compresses, thick gauze dressings attached to gauze bandages. A triangular bandage can be folded and used to cover a wound, or it can be used to hold a dressing or splint in

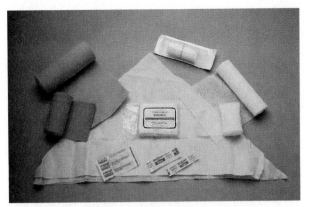

A bandage is any material used to wrap or cover any part of the body. It is often used to hold a dressing in place. Bandages include Band-Aids, triangular bandages, and roller bandages made of gauze or elastic material.

place. It can also be opened and used as a sling to support an injured arm, shoulder, or hand. A roller bandage is usually made of gauze or similar material. They come in widths from 1½ to 6 inches.

To apply a roller bandage, first raise the injured area above the

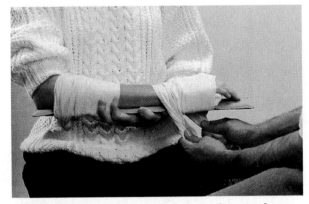

A folded triangular bandage can be used to secure a splint in place *(above)*. An open triangular bandage can be tied as a sling to support an injured arm *(right)*.

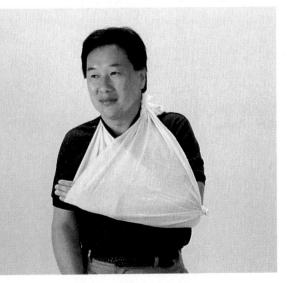

ROLLER BANDAGE

A roller bandage used to control bleeding is called a pressure bandage. To apply a pressure bandage ...

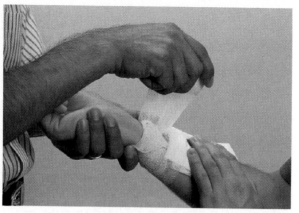

1 Start by securing the bandage over the dressing.

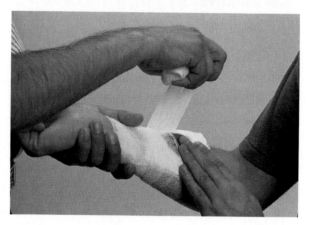

2 Use overlapping turns to cover the dressing completely.

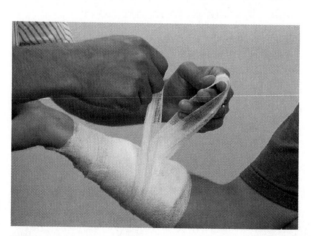

3 Tie or tape the bandage in place.

4 Check the fingers for warmth, color, and feeling.

level of the heart, if possible, to help slow bleeding. Secure one end of the bandage in place. Then wrap the bandage around the body part, using overlapping turns, covering the dressing, and extending several inches beyond the dressing at both ends. Tie or tape the bandage in place. If possible, do not cover the fingers or toes. Check them to see if they turn pale or blue or become cold. If they do, the bandage is too tight. Loosen it.

When a roller bandage is used to help control bleeding, it is commonly called a pressure bandage. This is because it can be applied snugly, keeping pressure over the wound. If blood soaks through bandages, put on more dressings and bandages. Do *not* remove blood-soaked ones.

Roller bandages can also be elastic. These are sometimes called Ace bandages. They are used to keep pressure on a part of the body, such as an arm or leg. They can control swelling and give support and are commonly used on joint injuries. Like other roller bandages, these elastic bandages are also available in assorted sizes.

Although an elastic bandage is very effective, it can create problems if it is applied so tightly that it restricts blood flow. Restricted blood flow is not only painful, it can cause tissue damage.

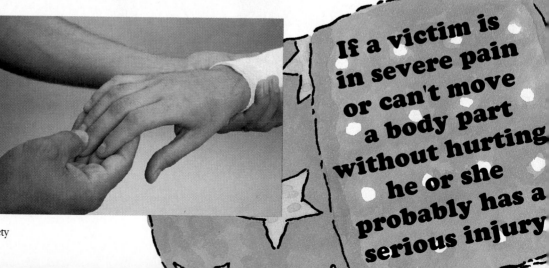

If a victim is in severe pain or can't move a body part without hurting he or she probably has a serious injury

The first step in using an elastic bandage is to select the correct size. This is determined by the area that you plan to wrap. A narrow bandage would be used to wrap a hand or wrist. A medium width bandage would be used for an arm or ankle. A wide bandage would be used to wrap a leg.

To begin the wrap, place the end of the bandage against the skin and use overlapping turns. Gently stretch the bandage as you continue the wrapping. The wrap should cover a long body section, like an arm or a calf, beginning at the point farthest from the heart. For a joint like a knee or ankle, use figure-eight turns to support the joint.

Be sure that the bandage is not too tight. Check the circulation of the limb beyond the bandage by noting changes in skin color and temperature.

CARING FOR SOFT TISSUE INJURIES

Most closed wounds, such as bruises, do not need special medical care. You can use direct pressure on the area to cut down bleeding under the skin. Raising the injured part helps reduce swelling.

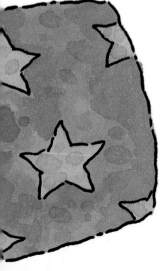

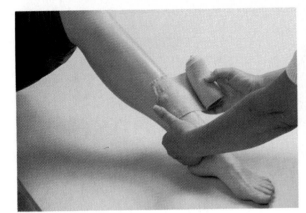

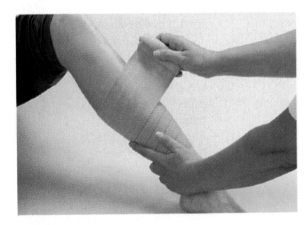

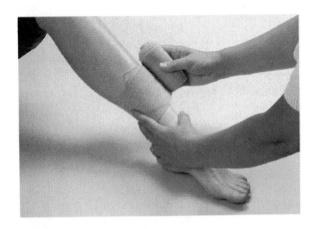

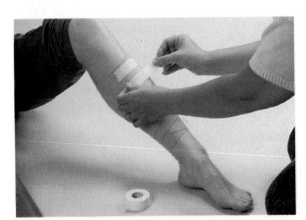

ELASTIC BANDAGE

Elastic bandages control swelling and give support for injuries such as sprains or strains. To apply an elastic bandage ...

Start at the point farthest from the heart.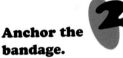

Anchor the bandage. **2**

Wrap the bandage using overlapping turns. **3**

Tape the bandage in place.

Blood and Disease Transmission

Disease transmission occurs when bacteria or viruses from one person enter the body of another person. If a victim has an infectious disease and is bleeding severely, there is an easy path for infection to travel. If you make contact with the victim's blood *and* you have a cut, scrape, or sore, a path exists for the infection to enter your body. This blood-to-blood contact provides an easy route for the infection to spread.

When you take action to control bleeding, it is also important to reduce the risk of infection. A properly equipped first aid kit can help you deal with a bleeding victim. Good personal hygiene practices, such as washing hands before and immediately after giving care, can also reduce the risk of disease transmission.

To reduce the risk of infection while you give care, you should do the following:

- Avoid being splashed by blood.
- Place a barrier between you and the victim's blood. This can be done by wearing disposable latex gloves and covering the wound with a dressing or plastic wrap.
- Cover any cuts, scrapes, or skin conditions you have.
- Wash your hands immediately after providing care, even if you wore gloves. Use a utility or rest room sink. Do not use a sink in a food preparation area.
- Avoid eating, drinking, and touching your mouth, eyes, or nose while providing care or before you wash your hands.
- Avoid touching objects that may have been contaminated with blood.
- Avoid handling any of your personal items, such as pens or combs, while providing care or before washing your hands.

These steps are safety precautions that can greatly reduce your risk of infection. Always give first aid in ways that protect both you and the victim from disease transmission.

Applying cold can help control pain and swelling. Always put a thin layer of cloth between the source of the cold and the victim's skin.

Some closed wounds, however, can be extremely serious. If a victim is in severe pain or can't move a body part without hurting, he or she probably has a serious injury. Ask yourself if the force that caused the injury was great enough to have caused serious damage. If you think it was, call for an ambulance at once. The victim may be bleeding internally and need professional medical help as soon as possible.

While you are waiting for the ambulance, help the victim rest in the most comfortable position.

SIGNALS OF INTERNAL BLEEDING

Tender, swollen, bruised, or hard areas of the body, such as the abdomen

Rapid, weak pulse

Skin that feels cool or moist or looks pale or bluish

Vomiting or coughing up blood

Excessive thirst

Becoming confused, faint, drowsy, or unconscious

Keep the victim from getting chilled or overheated. Reassure and comfort the victim.

A major open wound has serious tissue damage and severe bleeding. To care for a major open wound, you must act at once. Do *not* waste time washing the wound. Instead, begin by placing a dressing over the wound and applying direct pressure. If a sterile dressing isn't available, use any clean cloth, such as a towel, handkerchief, tie, or sock. If the victim is able to help, have him or her apply pressure to the wound. Use your own bare hand to apply pressure only as a last resort. Always try to put a barrier between yourself and a victim's blood. Keep a pair of disposable gloves handy, either in a first aid kit or in your car.

Next, elevate the wound. If possible, raise the injured area above the level of the heart. Then, apply a bandage snugly over the dressings to keep pressure on the wound. If the bleeding is still not controlled, use a pressure point. A pressure point is a spot on the body where you can squeeze the nearby artery against the bone underneath. This can slow or stop the flow of blood to the wound.

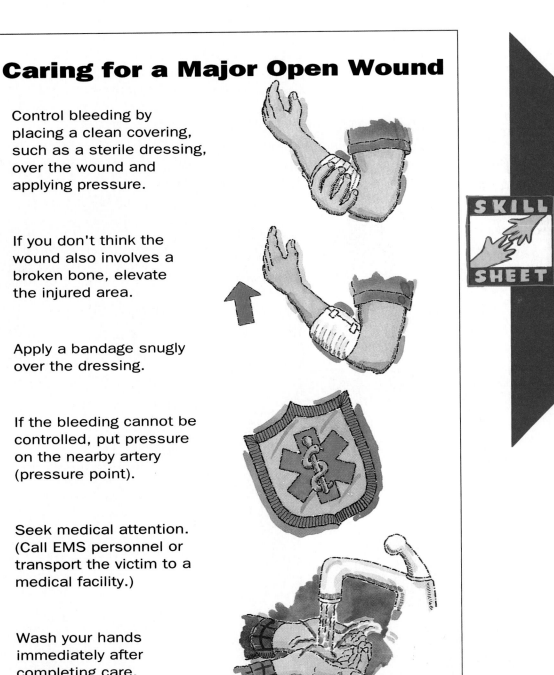

Caring for a Major Open Wound

Control bleeding by placing a clean covering, such as a sterile dressing, over the wound and applying pressure.

If you don't think the wound also involves a broken bone, elevate the injured area.

Apply a bandage snugly over the dressing.

If the bleeding cannot be controlled, put pressure on the nearby artery (pressure point).

Seek medical attention. (Call EMS personnel or transport the victim to a medical facility.)

Wash your hands immediately after completing care.

SKILL SHEET

If a Person is Bleeding...

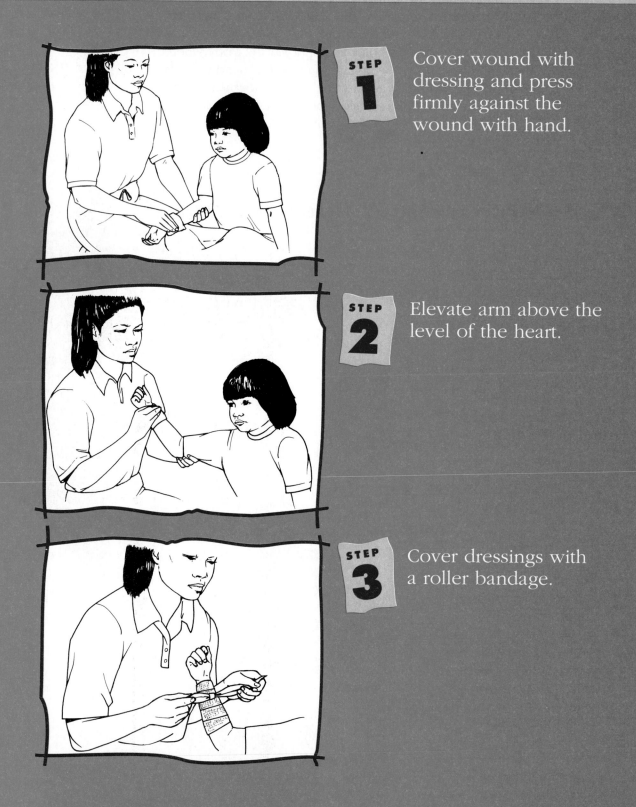

STEP 1 — Cover wound with dressing and press firmly against the wound with hand.

STEP 2 — Elevate arm above the level of the heart.

STEP 3 — Cover dressings with a roller bandage.

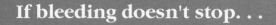

If bleeding doesn't stop. . .

STEP 4 Apply additional dressings.

STEP 5 Squeeze artery against bone.

If bleeding is from the leg, press with the heel of your hand where the leg bends at the hip.

SHOCK

Any severe bleeding can lead to a life-threatening condition called shock. Shock is a condition in which the circulatory system fails to deliver blood to all parts of the body. When the body's organs do not receive blood, they fail to function properly. This triggers a series of responses that produce specific signals known as shock. These responses are the body's attempt to maintain adequate blood flow.

When the body is healthy, the following three conditions are needed to maintain adequate blood flow:

• The heart must be working well.

• An adequate amount of blood must be circulating in the body.

• The blood vessels must be intact and able to adjust blood flow.

When someone is injured or suddenly becomes ill, these normal body functions may be interrupted. When the injury or illness is minor, the interruption is brief because the body is able to compensate quickly. With more severe injuries or illnesses, the body may be unable to adjust. When the body is unable to meet its demands for blood, shock occurs.

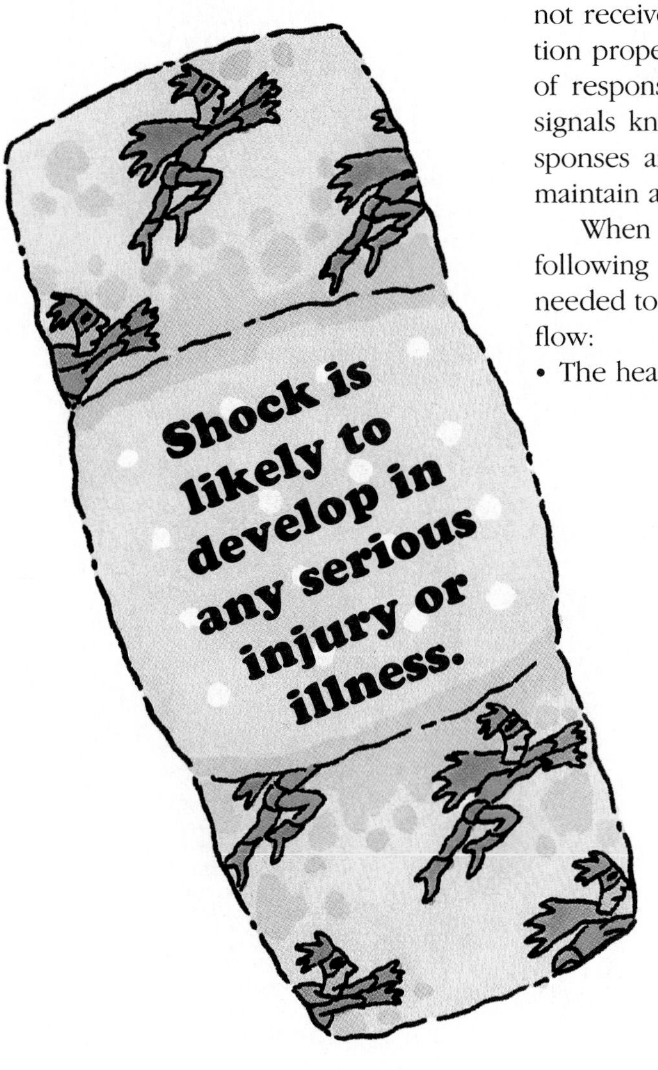

SIGNALS OF SHOCK

Although you might not always be able to determine the cause of shock, you should be able to recognize the following signals:

Restlessness or irritability (often the first indicator that the body is experiencing a significant problem)

Altered consciousness

Pale, cool, moist skin

Rapid breathing

Rapid pulse

For the heart to do its job properly, an adequate amount of blood must circulate within the body. The body can compensate for some decrease in the amount of blood. However, with severe injuries involving greater or more rapid loss

Shock is likely to develop in any serious injury or illness.

of blood, the body might not be able to adjust.

Any significant fluid loss, even as a result of diarrhea or vomiting, can cause shock. Such a decrease in body fluids affects the function of the heart. The heart eventually fails to beat properly, so the pulse becomes irregular or stops altogether.

Blood vessels act as pipelines to all parts of the body. For this circulation system to function properly, blood vessels must remain intact, preventing loss of blood. Normally, blood vessels can increase or decrease the flow of blood to different areas of the body. This ability ensures that blood reaches the areas of the body that need it most. Injuries or illnesses, especially those that affect the brain and spinal cord, can cause blood vessels to lose this ability to regulate the flow of blood. Blood vessels can also be affected if the nervous system is damaged by infections, drugs, or poisons.

If the heart is damaged, it can't pump blood properly. If blood vessels are damaged, the body can't adjust blood flow. Regardless of the cause, when the body does not get adequate blood, it also does not get adequate oxygen and the body goes into shock.

When shock occurs, the body attempts to adjust and send blood to the most important parts, such as the brain, heart, lungs, and kidneys. The body does this by reducing blood flow to the less important parts, such as the arms, legs, and skin. This is why the skin of a person in shock appears pale and feels cool. In the later stages of shock the skin, especially the lips and around the eyes, may appear blue from prolonged lack of oxygen.

CARING FOR SHOCK

Caring for shock involves the following simple steps:

Have the victim lie down. This is often the most comfortable position. Helping the victim rest comfortably is important because pain can intensify the body's stress and accelerate the progression of shock. Helping the victim rest in a more comfortable position may minimize any pain.

Control any external bleeding.

Help the victim maintain normal body temperature. If the victim is cool, try to cover him or her to avoid chilling.

Try to reassure the victim.

Elevate the legs about 12 inches unless you suspect head, neck, or back injuries or possible broken bones involving the hips or legs. If you are unsure of the victim's condition, leave him or her lying flat.

Do not give the victim anything to eat or drink, even though he or she is likely to be thirsty.

Call your local emergency number immediately. Shock can't be managed effectively by first aid alone. A victim of shock requires advanced medical care as soon as possible.

SHOCK: The Domino Effect

Any serious injury or illness will trigger a series of responses in the body that acts like a chain of falling dominoes. This condition is known as shock.

Shock is the body's natural attempt to keep oxygen-rich blood flowing to the most important organs, such as the brain, heart, and lungs. Without oxygen, these organs will fail to function properly. When the oxygen-deprived tissues of the arms and legs begin to die, the body sends blood back to them and away from the vital organs. As the brain is affected, the person becomes restless, drowsy, and eventually becomes unconscious. As the heart is affected, it beats irregularly, resulting in an irregular pulse. The heart's rhythm becomes chaotic and the heart fails to pump blood. There is no longer a pulse. When the heart stops, breathing stops. This chain of falling dominoes eventually results in death.

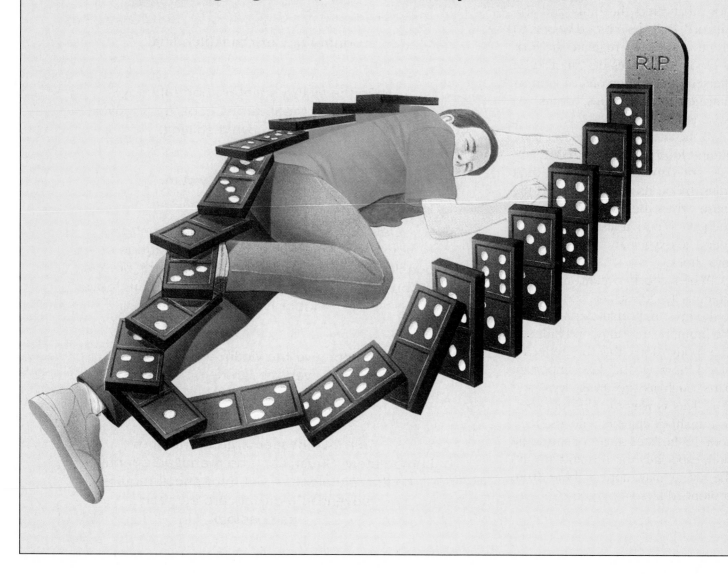

If part of the body has been torn or cut off, try to find the part and wrap it in sterile gauze or any clean material, such as a washcloth. Put the wrapped part in a plastic bag. Keep the part cool by placing the bag on ice, if possible, but do not freeze. Be sure the part is taken to the hospital with the victim. Doctors may be able to reattach it.

If an object, such as a knife or a piece of glass or metal, is impaled in a wound, *do not* remove it. Place several dressings around it to keep it from moving. Bandage the dressings in place around the object. If it is only a splinter in the skin, it can be removed with tweezers. After removing the splinter from the skin, wash the area. Then cover it to keep it clean. If the splinter is in the eye, you should not attempt to remove it. Call for an ambulance; the victim needs professional medical care.

Nose injuries are usually caused by a blow from a blunt object. The result is often a nosebleed. High blood pressure or changes in altitude can also cause nosebleeds. In most cases, you can control bleeding by having the victim sit with the head slightly forward while pinching the nostrils together. Other methods of controlling bleeding include applying an ice pack to the bridge of the nose or putting pressure on the upper lip just beneath the nose.

Your primary concern for injury to the mouth is to make sure the victim is able to breathe. Injuries to the mouth may cause breathing

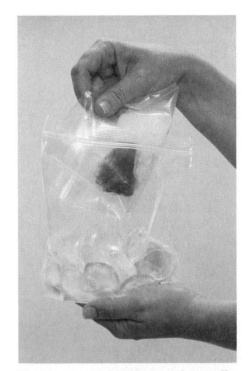

Wrap a severed body part in sterile gauze, put it in a plastic bag, and put the bag on ice. Be sure the part is taken to the hospital with the victim.

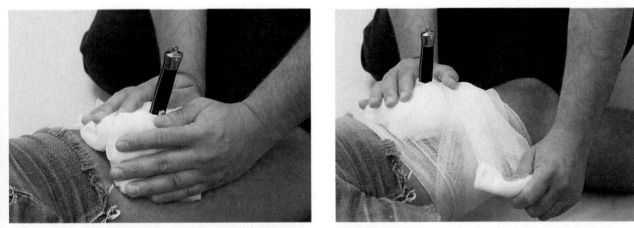

If an object is impaled in a wound, do not remove it. Bandage bulky dressings around the object to support it in place.

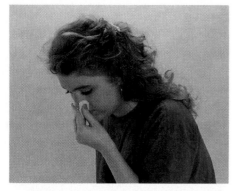

To control a nosebleed, have the victim lean forward and pinch the nostrils together until bleeding stops.

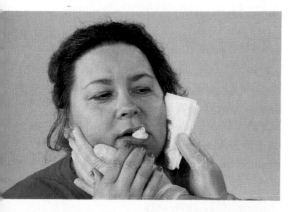

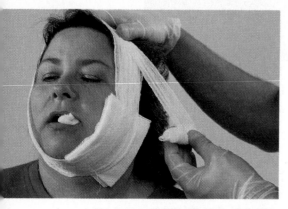

To control bleeding inside the cheek, place folded dressings inside the mouth against the wound (top). To control bleeding on the outside, use dressings to apply pressure directly to the wound and bandage so as not to restrict breathing (bottom).

problems if blood or loose teeth obstruct the airway.

If the victim is bleeding from the mouth and you do not suspect a serious head or spine injury, place the victim in a seated position with the head tilted slightly forward. This will allow any blood to drain from the mouth. If this position is not possible, place the victim on his or her side to allow blood to drain from the mouth.

For injuries that penetrate the lip, place a rolled dressing between the lip and the gum. You can place another dressing on the outer surface of the lip. If the tongue is bleeding, apply a dressing and direct pressure. Applying cold to the lips or tongue can help reduce swelling and ease pain.

If the injury knocked out one or more of the victim's teeth, control the bleeding and save any teeth so that they can be reinserted. To control the bleeding, roll a sterile dressing and insert it into the space left by the missing tooth. Have the victim bite down to maintain pressure.

For minor open wounds that don't bleed very much, such as

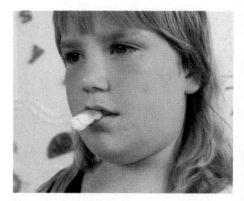

If a tooth is knocked out, place a sterile dressing directly in the space left by the tooth. Tell the victim to bite down.

scrapes, wash the wound thoroughly with soap and water. Put a sterile dressing over the wound and apply pressure for a few minutes, if necessary, to control any bleeding. When bleeding is controlled, take off the dressing and put an antibiotic ointment on the wound. Then cover the wound with a clean dressing and bandage.

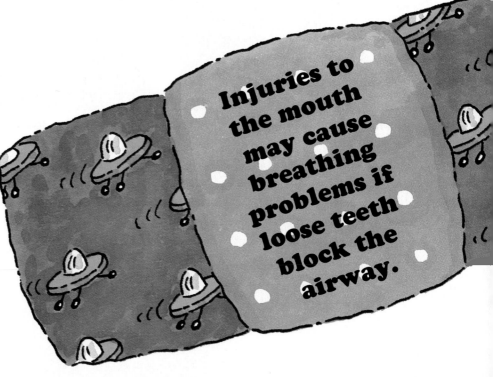

Injuries to the mouth may cause breathing problems if loose teeth block the airway.

NOW
SMILE!

Knocked-out teeth no longer have to lead to gapped smiles and bridgework. Most dentists can successfully replant a knocked-out tooth if they can do so quickly and if the tooth has been cared for properly.

Replanting a tooth is similar to replanting a tree. On each tooth, tiny root fibers attach to the jawbone to hold the tooth in place. Inside the tooth a canal filled with bundles of blood vessels and nerves runs from the tooth and into the jawbone and surrounding tissue.

When these fibers and tissues are torn from the socket, it is important for them to be replaced within an hour. Generally, the sooner the tooth is replanted, the better the chance it will survive. The knocked-out tooth must be handled carefully. Pick up the tooth by the chewing edge (crown), not the root. Do not rub or handle the root part of the tooth. If possible, place the tooth back in the socket in its normal position. Bite down gently and/or hold the tooth in position with a sterile gauze pad, a tissue, or a clean cloth. Be sure to see your dentist as soon as possible.

If you are unable to put the tooth back in its socket, preserve the tooth by placing it in a closed container of cool, fresh milk until it reaches the dentist. If milk is not available, use water.

A dentist or emergency room physician will clean the tooth. The tooth will then be placed back in the socket and secured with a special splint. The splint will hold the tooth stable while the fibers reattach to the jawbone. The bundles of blood vessels and nerves will grow back within 6 weeks.

Enamel (chewing edge)

Nerves and blood vessels

Root

REFERENCES

Bolgert, John, DDS, Executive Director, American Academy of Pediatric Dentists, Correspondence, January 1992.

Medford, Houck, DDS. Acute Care of An Avulsed Tooth. *Annals of Emergency Medicine* 11:559-61, 1982.

A puncture wound that penetrates the lung or the chest cavity surrounding the lung allows air to go in and out of the cavity.

Air from lung filling space around lung

Air from outside filling space around lung

BULLET PENETRATES CHEST CAVITY

cause severe bleeding or make breathing difficult. Because the chest and abdomen hold many organs important to life, injury to these areas can also cause a serious injury to the spine. Care for any life-threatening conditions first, then give any additional care that is needed.

The chest is the upper part of the trunk, formed by the ribs, breastbone, and spine. It contains the heart, lungs, and muscles that control breathing. A puncture wound to the chest can range from minor to life-threatening. Stab and gunshot wounds are examples of puncture injuries.

A forceful puncture to the chest may penetrate the rib cage. This allows air to freely pass in and out of the chest through the wound. This prevents the lungs from working normally. With each breath the victim takes, you may hear a sucking sound coming from the wound. This is the main signal of a penetrating chest injury called a sucking chest wound. The penetrating object can also injure structures within the chest, including the lungs, heart, or major arteries or veins.

Most injuries to the chest and abdomen are only minor cuts, scratches, and bruises. Sometimes, more serious injuries can occur, such as those resulting from motor vehicle crashes, falls, and stab and bullet wounds. These injuries can

A special dressing with one loose corner keeps air from the wound when breathing in and allows air to escape when breathing out.

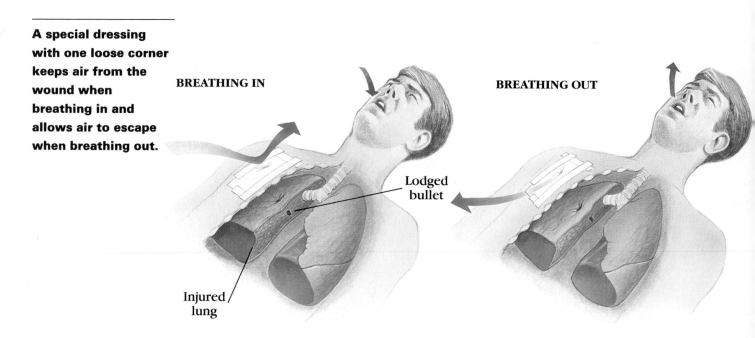

BREATHING IN

BREATHING OUT

Lodged bullet

Injured lung

Without care, the victim's condition will quickly get worse. One or both lungs will fail to work properly and breathing will become more difficult. Your number one concern is the victim's breathing problem.

To care for a sucking chest wound, cover the wound with a dressing that does not allow air to pass through it. A plastic bag, a plastic or latex glove, or a piece of plastic wrap or aluminum foil folded several times and placed over the wound will work if a special sterile dressing is not available. Tape the dressing in place, except for one corner that should stay loose. If none of these materials are available, use a folded cloth. Give any other care that is necessary.

The abdomen is the soft area of the belly, below the chest. Because the abdomen is not protected by any bones, it is easily injured. A forceful blow to the abdomen or a fall from a height can cause severe bleeding inside the body. If you suspect severe internal bleeding, keep the victim lying flat and watch for signals of internal bleeding. Bending the knees and hips slightly may make the victim more comfortable. A folded blanket or a pillow can be placed under the knees to support the legs in this position. If movement of the legs causes pain, leave the victim lying flat.

Sometimes a severe blow or penetrating injury to the abdomen can cause organs to be exposed or protrude. In this case, carefully position the victim on his or her back. Do not apply any pressure to the organs and do not attempt to push the organs back inside. Remove any clothing from around the wound and apply moist, sterile dressings or a clean cloth loosely over the wound. Use warm tap water to moisten the dressings.

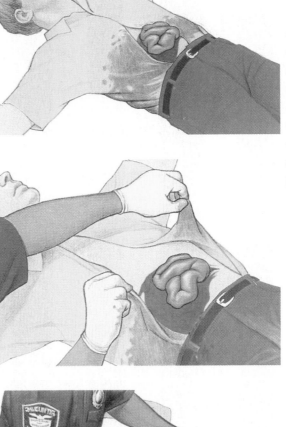

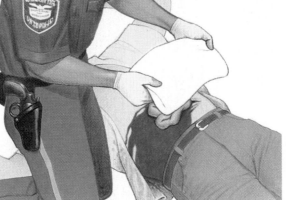

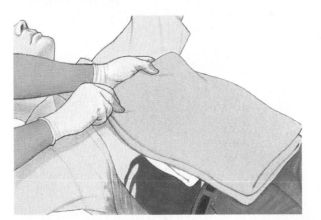

Wounds that break through the abdomen can cause the organs to push out. Carefully remove clothing from around the wound. Cover the organs with a moist sterile or clean dressing and cover the dressing with plastic wrap. Place a folded towel or other cloth over the dressing to keep the organs warm.

BURNS

Burns are a specific type of soft tissue injury.

Burns caused by heat are the most common. Certain chemicals, however, can also cause burns. Electrical current can burn the body internally and externally. Radiation from the sun can cause sunburn. A burn first destroys the top layer of skin. If it continues to burn, it injures or destroys the second

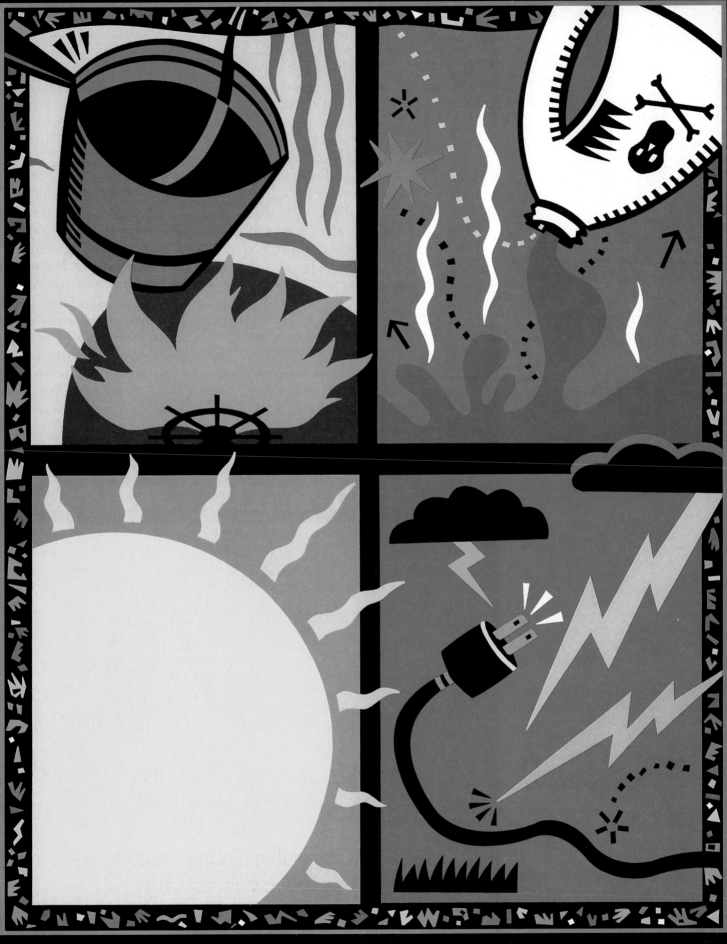

A critical burn can be life-threatening and needs immediate medical attention.

layer of skin. When burns break the skin, they can cause infection and loss of fluid from the body and can damage the body's ability to control its temperature. Deep burns can also damage the victim's ability to breathe.

The severity of a burn depends on the temperature of whatever caused the burn and the length of time the victim is exposed to it. The severity is also affected by the burn's location on the body, the size of the burn, and the victim's age and medical condition.

You can describe burns by their cause—heat, electricity, chemicals, and radiation—or by their depth. The deeper the burn, the more severe it is.

A burn that involves only the top layer of skin is the least severe. The skin is red and dry and the burn hurts. These burns usually heal in 5 to 6 days and don't leave scars.

Deeper burns are also red. They have blisters that may open and weep clear fluid. The burned skin may look blotchy. These burns are usually painful and the area often swells.

Some burns destroy all the layers of skin and the tissues underneath. They can even destroy bones. These burns look brown or blackish. The tissues underneath may appear white. These burns can sometimes be surprisingly pain-free because nerve endings have been destroyed. These burns are critical.

A critical burn needs immediate medical attention. Critical burns can be life-threatening. It isn't always easy to tell how severe a burn is right after it has happened. Call

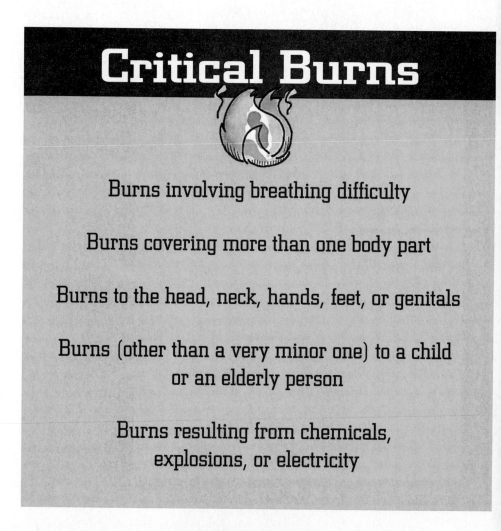

Critical Burns

Burns involving breathing difficulty

Burns covering more than one body part

Burns to the head, neck, hands, feet, or genitals

Burns (other than a very minor one) to a child or an elderly person

Burns resulting from chemicals, explosions, or electricity

for an ambulance immediately if a burn victim is having trouble breathing or has burns on more than one part of the body. Call if the victim has burns on the head, neck, back, hands, feet, or genitals. Call for any burns caused by chemicals, explosions, or electricity.

Burns caused by flames or hot grease usually need medical attention, especially if the victim is a child or an elderly person. Burns caused by hot liquid or flames that contact clothing also are serious, since the clothing keeps the heat in contact with the skin. Some fabrics even melt and stick to the skin. All these burns may look minor at first, but they can continue to get worse.

CARE FOR BURNS

To care for a burn, follow these basic steps. First, stop the burning. For example, you may have to put out flames that have caught clothing. Next, use water to cool the burned area. Don't use ice except on minor burns, such as a burned finger from touching a hot stove.

After cooling the burned area for several minutes, cover the burn with dry, clean dressings to help prevent infection. Bandage loosely—don't put any pressure on the burn. Don't put any kind of ointment on a burn unless it is a very minor burn. Ointment may seal in heat and doesn't do much to relieve pain. Don't use other home remedies; they can cause infection. Don't break blisters; keeping the skin unbroken helps prevent infection.

For minor burns and burns with open blisters that aren't bad enough to need medical care, wash the area with soap and water. Keep it clean. Put on an antibiotic ointment, such as Neosporin. Watch for signals of infection.

Lay a victim of severe burns down unless he or she is having

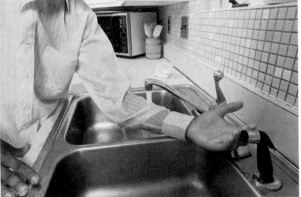

To care for a burn, first stop the burning.

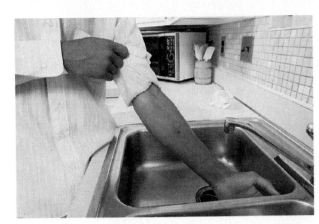

Cool the burned area with large amounts of cool water.

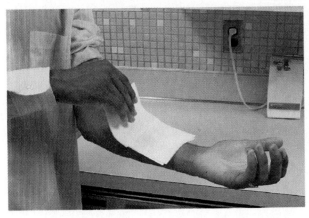

Then cover the burn with dry, clean dressings to help prevent infection.

BURNS

Superficial Burn
(First Degree)

Involves only the top layer of skin. The skin is red and dry, and the burn is usually painful. The area may swell. Most sunburns are superficial burns. Superficial burns usually heal in 5 to 6 days without permanent scarring.

Partial-thickness Burn
(Second Degree)

Involves the top layers of skin. The skin is red and has blisters that may open and weep clear fluid, making the skin appear wet. The burned skin may appear mottled. These burns are usually painful, and the area often swells. The burn usually heals in 3 to 4 weeks. Scarring may occur.

Full-thickness Burn
(Third Degree)

Destroys all layers of skin and any or all of the underlying structures—fat, muscles, bones and nerves. These burns look brown or black (charred) with the tissues underneath sometimes appearing white. They can either be extremely painful or relatively painless if the burn destroys the nerve endings.

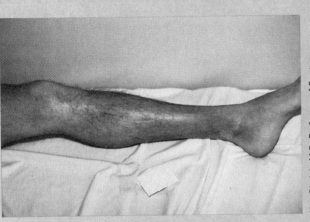

Alan Dimick, M.D. Professor of Surgery, Director of UAB Burn Center

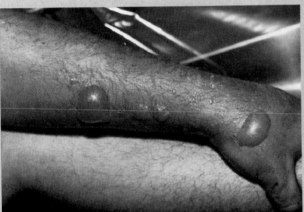

Alan Dimick, M.D. Professor of Surgery, Director of UAB Burn Center

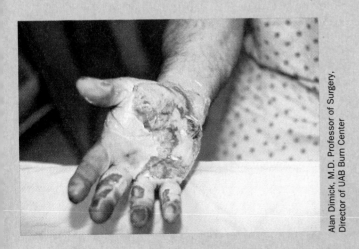

Alan Dimick, M.D. Professor of Surgery, Director of UAB Burn Center

CARE FOR BURNS

The care for burns involves the following three basic steps:

1 Stop the Burning.
Put out flames or remove the victim from the source of the burn.

2 Cool the Burn.
Use large amounts of cool water to cool the burned area. Do not use ice or ice water other than on small superficial burns. Ice causes body heat loss. Use whatever resources are available—tub, shower, or garden hose, for example. You can apply soaked towels, sheets, or other wet cloths to a burned face or other areas that cannot be immersed. Be sure to keep the cloths cool by adding more water.

3 Cover the Burn.
Use dry, sterile dressings or a clean cloth. Loosely bandage them in place. Covering the burn helps keep out air and reduces pain. Covering the burn also helps prevent infection. If the burn covers a large area of the body, cover it with clean, dry sheets or other cloth.

FYI

Within Striking Distance

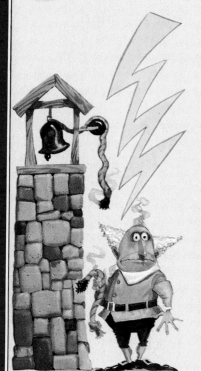

In medieval times, people believed that ringing church bells would get rid of lightning during thunderstorms. It was an unfortunate superstition for bell ringers. In 33 years, lightning struck 386 church steeples and 103 bell ringers died.[1]

Church bell ringers have dropped off the list of people most likely to be struck during a thunderstorm, but lightning strikes remain very dangerous. Lightning causes more deaths each year in the United States than any other weather hazard, including blizzards, hurricanes, floods, tornadoes, earthquakes, and volcanic eruptions. The National Weather Service estimates that lightning kills nearly 100 people every year and injures about 300 others. Lightning occurs when particles of water, ice, and air moving inside storm clouds lose electrons. Eventually, the cloud becomes divided into layers of positive and negative particles. Most electrical current remains inside the cloud. Sometimes, however, the negative charge flashes toward the ground, which has a positive charge. An electrical current snakes back and forth between the cloud and the ground many times in the seconds that we see a flash crackle down from the sky. Anything tall—a tower, a tree, or a person—becomes a path for the electrical current.

Traveling at speeds up to 300 miles per second, a lightning strike can hurl a person through the air. It can burn clothes off and can sometimes cause the heart to stop beating. The most severe lightning strikes carry up to 50 million volts of electricity, enough to serve 13,000 homes. Lightning can "flash" over a person's body, or it can travel through blood vessels and nerves to reach the ground.

Besides burns, lightning can also cause nervous system damage, broken bones, and loss of hearing or eyesight. Victims sometimes act confused and suffer memory loss. They may describe what happened as getting hit on the head or hearing an explosion.

Use common sense during thunderstorms. If you see a storm approaching in the distance, don't wait until you are soaked to seek shelter. If a thunderstorm threatens, the National Weather Service advises you to—

- Go inside a large building or home.
- Go inside a car and roll up the windows.
- Stop swimming or boating as soon as you see or hear a storm since water conducts electricity.
- Stay away from the telephone, except in an emergency.
- Stay away from telephone poles and tall trees if you are caught outside.
- Stay off hilltops; try to crouch down in a ravine or valley.
- Stay away from farm equipment and small metal vehicles, such as motorcycles, bicycles, and golf carts.
- Avoid wire fences, clotheslines, metal pipes and rails, and other conductors.
- Stay several yards apart if you are in a group.

REFERENCES
1. Kessler, Edwin. *The Thunderstorm in Human Affairs*, Norman, OK: University of Oklahoma, 1983.

2. Randall, Teri. *The Chicago Tribune*, Section 2D. August 13, 1989, p. 1.

trouble breathing. Raise burned areas above the level of the heart, if possible. Burn victims chill easily, so protect the victim from drafts.

SPECIAL KINDS OF BURNS

Chemical burns can happen both in the workplace and at home. Certain chemicals used in laboratory work and other jobs can cause severe burns if they contact the skin or eyes; so can various household products, such as cleansers, lawn and garden sprays, paint removers, and household bleach. The stronger the chemical and the longer the contact, the worse the burn. The chemical continues to burn as long as it is on the skin. You must remove the chemical from the skin as quickly as possible and call for an ambulance. If possible, have someone call while you care for the victim.

For chemical burns to the skin or eyes, flush the burn with large amounts of cool running water un-

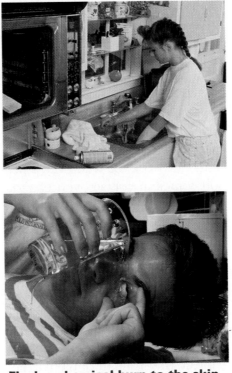

Flush a chemical burn to the skin *(top)* or eyes *(bottom)* with cool running water until the ambulance arrives.

Flush a chemical burn to the skin or eyes with large amounts of cool running water.

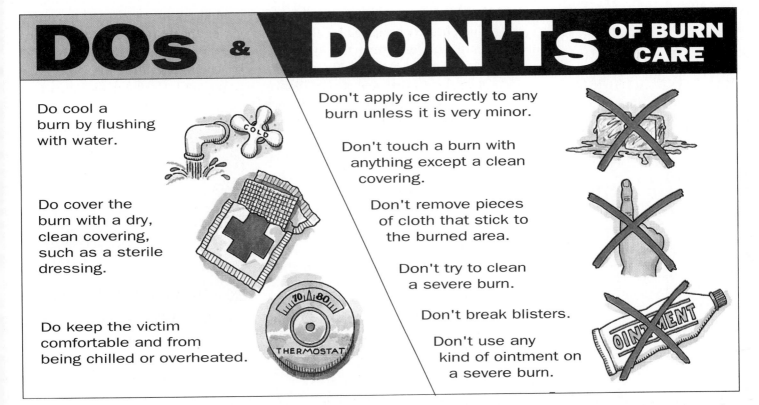

DOs & DON'TS OF BURN CARE

Do cool a burn by flushing with water.

Do cover the burn with a dry, clean covering, such as a sterile dressing.

Do keep the victim comfortable and from being chilled or overheated.

Don't apply ice directly to any burn unless it is very minor.

Don't touch a burn with anything except a clean covering.

Don't remove pieces of cloth that stick to the burned area.

Don't try to clean a severe burn.

Don't break blisters.

Don't use any kind of ointment on a severe burn.

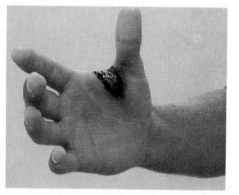

An electrical burn may severely damage underlying tissues.

Never go near a victim you think has been injured by electricity until you are sure the power has been turned off.

til the ambulance arrives. Have the victim take off any clothes with the chemical on them, if possible. If only one eye has been exposed to the chemical, flush the affected eye from the nose outward to prevent washing the chemical into the unaffected eye.

Electrical burns can happen at home, at work, or wherever a person comes in contact with electricity. Sources of electricity include power lines, lightning, defective electrical household equipment, and unprotected electrical outlets. Coming in contact with one of these sources can send electricity through the body. The severity of a burn depends on how long the body is in contact with the electric current, the strength of the current, the type of current, and the direction it takes through the body. These burns are often deep. The victim may have two wounds, one where the current entered the body and one where it left. These wounds may look minor, but the tissues beneath them may be severely damaged.

Never go near a victim you think has been injured by electricity until you are sure the power is turned off. *If a power line is down, wait for the fire department and/or the power company.* If there are people in a car with a downed wire across it, tell them not to move and to stay in the car.

With an electrical burn, the burn itself will not be the major problem. Check breathing and pulse if the victim is unconscious. Check for other injuries, such as possible fractures. The victim may have a spinal injury, so do not move him or her. Cover an electrical burn with a dry, sterile dressing, but do not cool the burn. Keep the victim from getting chilled.

Radiation from the sun and other sources can cause painful burns that may blister. Cool the burn. A doctor or pharmacist can tell you about products to put on mild burns such as minor sunburn. The victim can protect the burn from further damage by staying out of the sun. If you are going to be spending time in direct sun, it is wise to wear a protective lotion or cream.

People are unlikely to be exposed to other types of radiation unless they work in special settings. If they do, they are trained to prevent exposure.

Most of the burns you will have to deal with will be minor ones. Cool them, put on an antibiotic ointment, and cover them to prevent infection. If you encounter a victim with a more severe burn, stop the burning, and cover the burned area to prevent infection. Keep the victim from getting chilled and call your local emergency number. If the burn was caused by electricity, check for life-threatening conditions and other complications, such as fractures. Cover the burned area with a dry dressing. If the victim was burned by chemicals, flush the burn with water until the ambulance arrives.

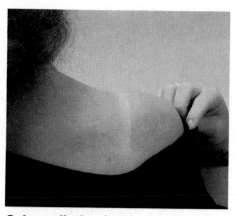

Solar radiation burns can be painful.

TOO MUCH OF A GOOD THING

Contrary to some beliefs, tan is not in. Although brief exposure to the sun causes your skin to produce the vitamin D necessary for the healthy formation of bones, long exposure can cause problems, such as sunburn, skin cancer, and early aging—a classic case of too much of a good thing being bad.

There are two kinds of ultraviolet (UV) light rays to be concerned about. Ultraviolet beta rays (UVB) are the burn-producing rays that more commonly cause skin cancer. These are the rays that damage the skin's surface and cause you to blister and peel. The other rays, ultraviolet alpha rays (UVA), have been heralded by tanning salons as "safe rays." Tanning salons claim to use lights that only emit UVA rays. Although UVA rays may not appear as harmful as UVB rays to the skin's surface, they more readily penetrate the deeper layers of the skin. This increases the risk of skin cancer, skin aging, eye damage, and changes that may alter the skin's ability to fight disease.

How do you get enough sun without getting too much? First avoid exposure to the sun between 10:00 a.m. and 2:00 p.m. UV rays are most harmful during this period. Second, wear proper clothing. Third, if you are going to be exposed to the sun, protect your skin and eyes.

Commercial sunscreens come in various strengths. The American Academy of Dermatology recommends

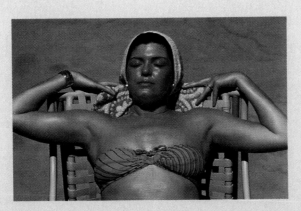

year-round sun protection including use of a high Sun Protection Factor (SPF) sunscreen for everyone, but particularly for people who are fair-skinned and sunburn easily. The Food and Drug Administration (FDA) has evaluated SPF readings and recognizes values between 2 and 15. It has not been determined whether sunscreens with ratings over 15 offer additional protection.

You should apply sunscreen 15 to 30 minutes before exposure to the sun and reapply it often (every 60 to 90 minutes). Swimmers should use sunscreens labeled as water-resistant and reapply them as described on the label.

Your best bet is to use a sunscreen that claims to protect against both UVB and UVA rays. Carefully check the label to determine the protection a product offers. Some products only offer protection against UVB rays.

It is equally important to protect your eyes from sun damage. Sunglasses are a sunscreen for your eyes and provide important protection from UV rays. Be sure to wear sunglasses that are labeled with their UV-absorbing ability. Ophthalmologists recommend sunglasses that have a UV absorption of at least 90 percent.

The next time the sun beckons, put on some sunscreen and your sunglasses, go outside, and have a great time.

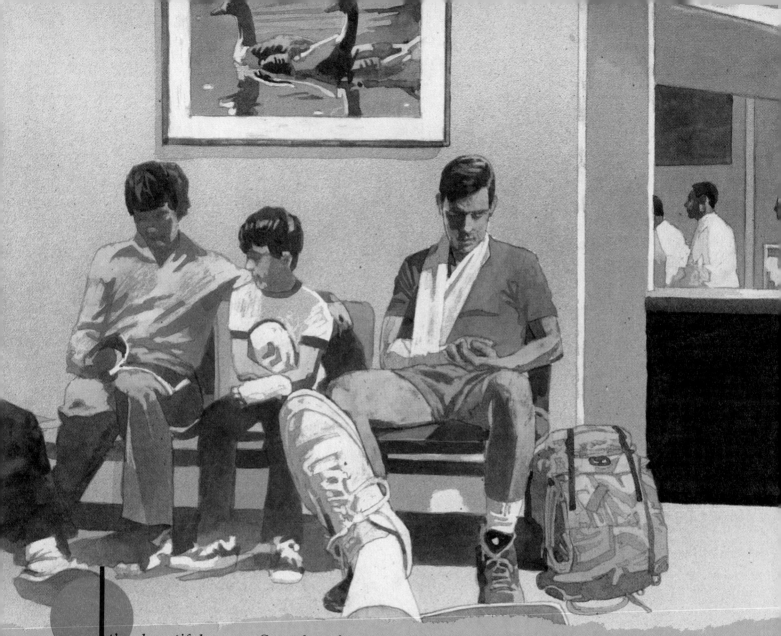

I t's a beautiful, sunny Saturday afternoon, and where are you? In the hospital emergency room, that's where, with a knee hurting so bad you had to borrow crutches to get there. Maybe it's time to give up the weekend athletics. You pass the time waiting your turn and watching the other visitors. They come in all ages and sizes. Here's a 14-year-old football player complete with anxious parents and

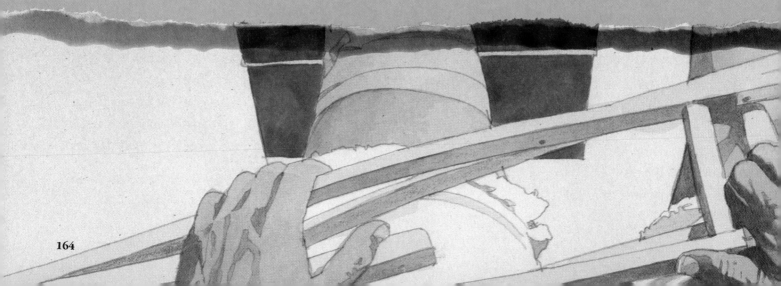

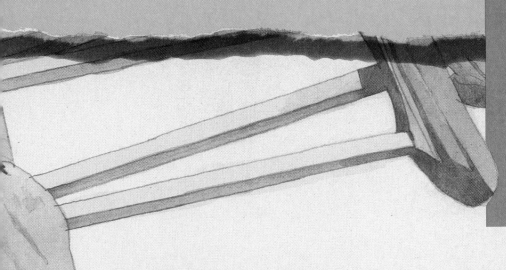

INJURY TO MUSCLES, BONES, AND JOINTS

a throbbing ankle. Watching TV is the forty-something would-be rock climber—who couldn't. An ambulance pulls up and an ashen, gray-haired victim with legs splinted is wheeled by the waiting room. What do each of these people have in common? Each has some sort of injury to a muscle, bone, or joint.

Injuries to muscles, bones, and joints happen often. They happen to all ages. They happen at home, at work, and at play. They are painful and they make life difficult. A person may fall and bruise the muscles of one leg, making walking painful. Equipment may fall on a worker and break bones. A person bracing one hand against the dashboard in an automobile crash may injure the bones at the shoulder and disable the arm. A skier may fall and twist a leg, tearing muscles and making it impossible to stand or move.

Injuries like these are almost always painful, but they are rarely life-threatening. If they aren't recog-nized and cared for, however, they can cause serious problems and even disable the victim.

The body's skeleton is made up of bones and muscles and the ten-dons and ligaments that connect them. Together, they give the body shape and stability. Bones and mus-cles connect to form various parts of the body. They work together to allow the body to move.

Muscles are soft tissues. The body has over 600 muscles, most of them attached to bones by strong tissues called tendons. Unlike other soft tissues, muscles are able to shorten and lengthen—contract and relax. This contracting and re-laxing is what makes the body move. The brain directs the mus-cles to move through the spinal cord, a pathway of nerves in the spine. Tiny jolts of electricity called electrical impulses travel through the nerves to the muscles. They cause the muscles to contract. When the muscles contract, they pull at the bones, causing motion at a joint.

BONES

Over 200 bones in various sizes and shapes form the skeleton. The skeleton protects many of the organs inside the body.

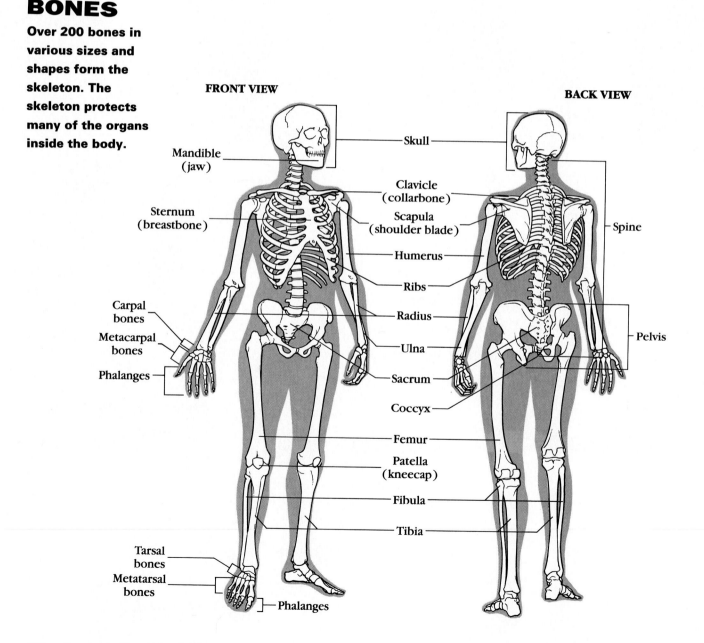

FRONT VIEW

BACK VIEW

Skull

Mandible (jaw)

Clavicle (collarbone)

Scapula (shoulder blade)

Sternum (breastbone)

Humerus

Ribs

Carpal bones

Radius

Metacarpal bones

Ulna

Phalanges

Sacrum

Coccyx

Spine

Pelvis

Femur

Patella (kneecap)

Fibula

Tibia

Tarsal bones

Metatarsal bones

Phalanges

Injuries to the brain, the spinal cord, or the nerves can affect muscle control. When nerves lose control of muscles, it is called paralysis. When a muscle is injured, a nearby muscle often takes over for the injured one.

Approximately 200 bones in various sizes and shapes form the skeleton. The skeleton protects many of the organs inside the body. Bones are hard and dense. Because they are strong and rigid, they are not injured easily. Bones have a

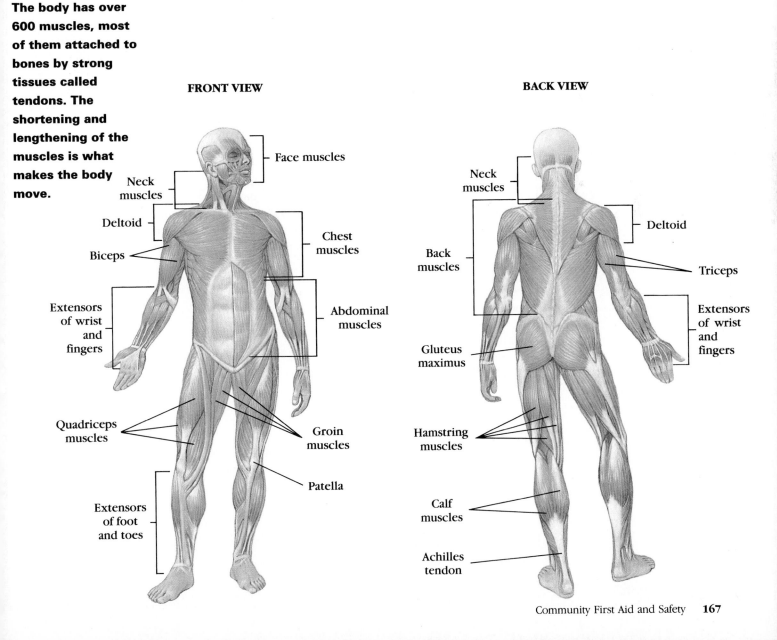

Brain

To brain

Connecting nerve cell

Motor nerve

Spinal cord

Sensory nerve

Messages are sent to and from the brain by way of nerves.

MUSCLES

The body has over 600 muscles, most of them attached to bones by strong tissues called tendons. The shortening and lengthening of the muscles is what makes the body move.

FRONT VIEW

- Face muscles
- Neck muscles
- Deltoid
- Biceps
- Chest muscles
- Abdominal muscles
- Extensors of wrist and fingers
- Quadriceps muscles
- Groin muscles
- Patella
- Extensors of foot and toes

BACK VIEW

- Neck muscles
- Back muscles
- Deltoid
- Triceps
- Extensors of wrist and fingers
- Gluteus maximus
- Hamstring muscles
- Calf muscles
- Achilles tendon

The Breaking Point

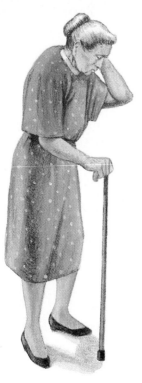

Osteoporosis is a bone disorder usually discovered after a person reaches the age of 60. It affects 30 percent of people over age 65. It strikes one out of four American women and occurs less frequently in men. Fair-skinned women with ancestors from northern Europe, the British Isles, Japan, or China are more likely to develop osteoporosis. Inactive people are also more susceptible to it.

Osteoporosis occurs when the calcium content of bone decreases. Normal bones are hard, dense tissues that endure great stresses. Calcium is a key to bone growth, development, and repair. When the calcium content of bones decreases, bones become frail and less dense. They are less able to repair the normal damage they incur. This leaves bones, especially hips, back, and wrists, more prone to fractures. These fractures may occur with only a little force. Some even occur without force. The victim may be taking a walk or washing dishes when the fracture occurs.

Osteoporosis can begin as early as age 30. The amount of calcium a person absorbs from his or her diet declines with age, making calcium intake more important.

Building strong bones before age 35 is the key to preventing osteoporosis. Calcium and exercise are necessary to bone building. Three to four daily servings of low-fat dairy products should provide enough calcium. Vitamin D also is necessary because it helps calcium. Exposure to sunshine enables the body to make vitamin D. Dark-skinned and elderly people need more exposure to the sun. People who do not receive adequate exposure to the sun need to eat foods that contain vitamin D. The best sources are vitamin-fortified milk and fatty fish, such as tuna, salmon, and eel.

People who do not take in adequate calcium can obtain calcium supplements. Some are combined with vitamin D. However, before taking a calcium supplement, consult a physician. Many highly advertised calcium supplements are ineffec-

tive because they do not dissolve in the body.

Exercise seems to increase bone density and the activity of bone-building cells. Regular exercise may reduce the rate of bone loss by promoting new bone formation. It may also stimulate the skeletal system to repair itself. An effective exercise program, such as aerobics, jogging, or walking, involves the weight-bearing muscles of the legs.

If you have any questions about your health and osteoporosis, consult your physician. Take care of your bones and don't let osteoporosis get you down.

rich supply of blood and nerves. Bone injuries can bleed and they usually hurt. If the injury is not cared for, the bleeding can become life-threatening. Bones weaken with age. Children have more flexible bones than adults; their bones break less easily. Older adults have more brittle bones. Sometimes they break surprisingly easily. This gradual weakening of bones is called osteoporosis.

A joint is formed by the ends of two or more bones coming together at one place. Most joints allow the body to move at that spot. The bones at a joint are held together by strong, tough bands called ligaments. All joints have a normal range of movement—an area in which they can move freely without too much stress or strain. When joints are forced beyond this range, ligaments stretch and tear.

The four basic types of injuries to muscles, bones, and joints are fractures, dislocations, strains, and sprains. They happen in a variety of ways. A fracture is a complete break, a chip, or a crack in a bone. It can be caused by a fall, a blow,

and sometimes even a twisting movement.

Fractures are open or closed. An open fracture involves an open wound. It occurs when an arm or a leg bends in such a way that bone

Fractures include chipped or cracked bones and bones broken all the way through.

ends tear through the skin. An object that goes into the skin, such as a bullet, and breaks a bone can also cause an open fracture. In a closed fracture the skin is not broken. Closed fractures are more common. Open fractures are more dangerous; they carry a risk of infection and severe bleeding. In general, fractures are life-threatening only if they involve breaks in large bones such as the thigh, sever an artery, or affect breathing. Since you can't always tell if a person has a fracture, you should consider the cause of the injury. A fall from a height or a motor vehicle accident, for instance, is a signal that a fracture is possible.

Dislocations are usually more obvious than fractures. A dislocation is the movement of a bone at a joint away from its normal position. This movement is usually caused by a violent force tearing the ligaments

A typical joint consists of two or more bones held together by ligaments.

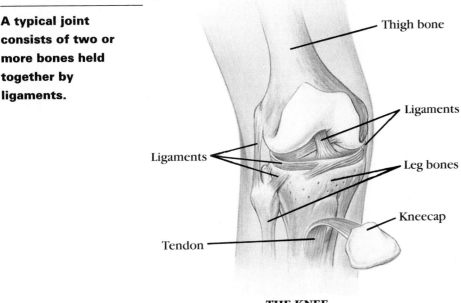

Thigh bone

Ligaments

Ligaments

Leg bones

Kneecap

Tendon

THE KNEE

that hold the bones in place. When a bone is moved out of place, the joint no longer functions. The displaced bone end often forms a bump, a ridge, or a hollow that doesn't normally exist.

A sprain is the tearing of ligaments at a joint. Mild sprains may swell but usually heal quickly. The victim might not feel much pain and is active again soon. If a victim ignores the signals of swelling and pain and becomes active too soon, the joint won't heal properly and will remain weak. There is a good chance it will become reinjured, only this time more severely. A severe sprain can also involve a fracture or dislocation of the bones at the joint. The joints most easily injured are at the ankle, knee, wrist, and fingers.

A strain is a stretching and tearing of muscles or tendons. Strains are often caused by lifting something heavy or working a muscle too hard. They usually involve the muscles in the neck, back, or thigh or the back of the lower leg. Some strains can reoccur, especially in the neck or back.

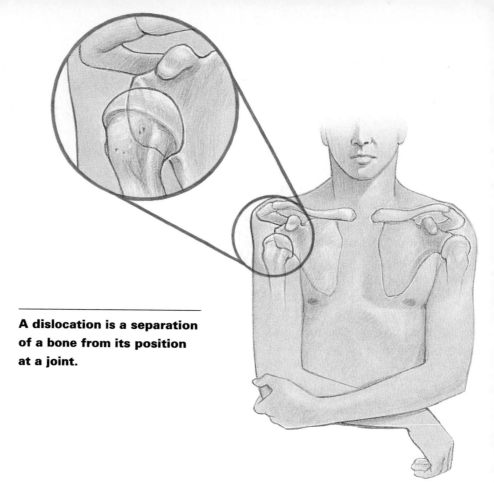

A dislocation is a separation of a bone from its position at a joint.

How can you tell how bad the injury is to a muscle, bone, or joint? Often you can't. Sometimes an x ray is needed to determine the extent of the injury. Certain signals, however, can give you a clue regarding whether the injury is severe.

One of the most common signals is pain. The injured area may be painful to touch and to move. The area may be swollen and red or bruised. The area may be twisted or strangely bent. It may have abnormal lumps, ridges, and hollows.

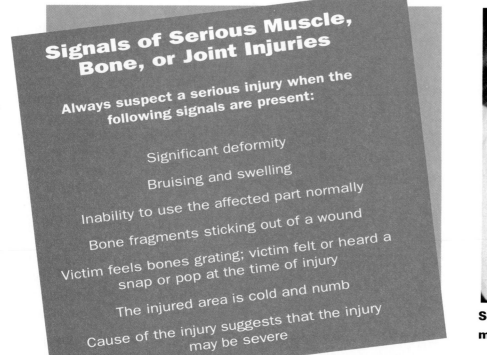

Signals of Serious Muscle, Bone, or Joint Injuries

Always suspect a serious injury when the following signals are present:

Significant deformity

Bruising and swelling

Inability to use the affected part normally

Bone fragments sticking out of a wound

Victim feels bones grating; victim felt or heard a snap or pop at the time of injury

The injured area is cold and numb

Cause of the injury suggests that the injury may be severe

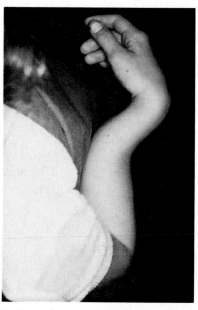

COSF-Boston

Serious bone or joint injuries may appear deformed.

Whether an injury is a sprain or strain is often confusing. A sprain is the partial or complete stretching or tearing of the special soft tissue bands that hold bones together at a joint, called ligaments. A strain is a stretching or tearing of muscles or the strong fibers that attach muscle to bone, called tendons. In short, injuries to joints are usually sprains; injuries to the soft tissue between joints, the muscles and tendons, are strains.

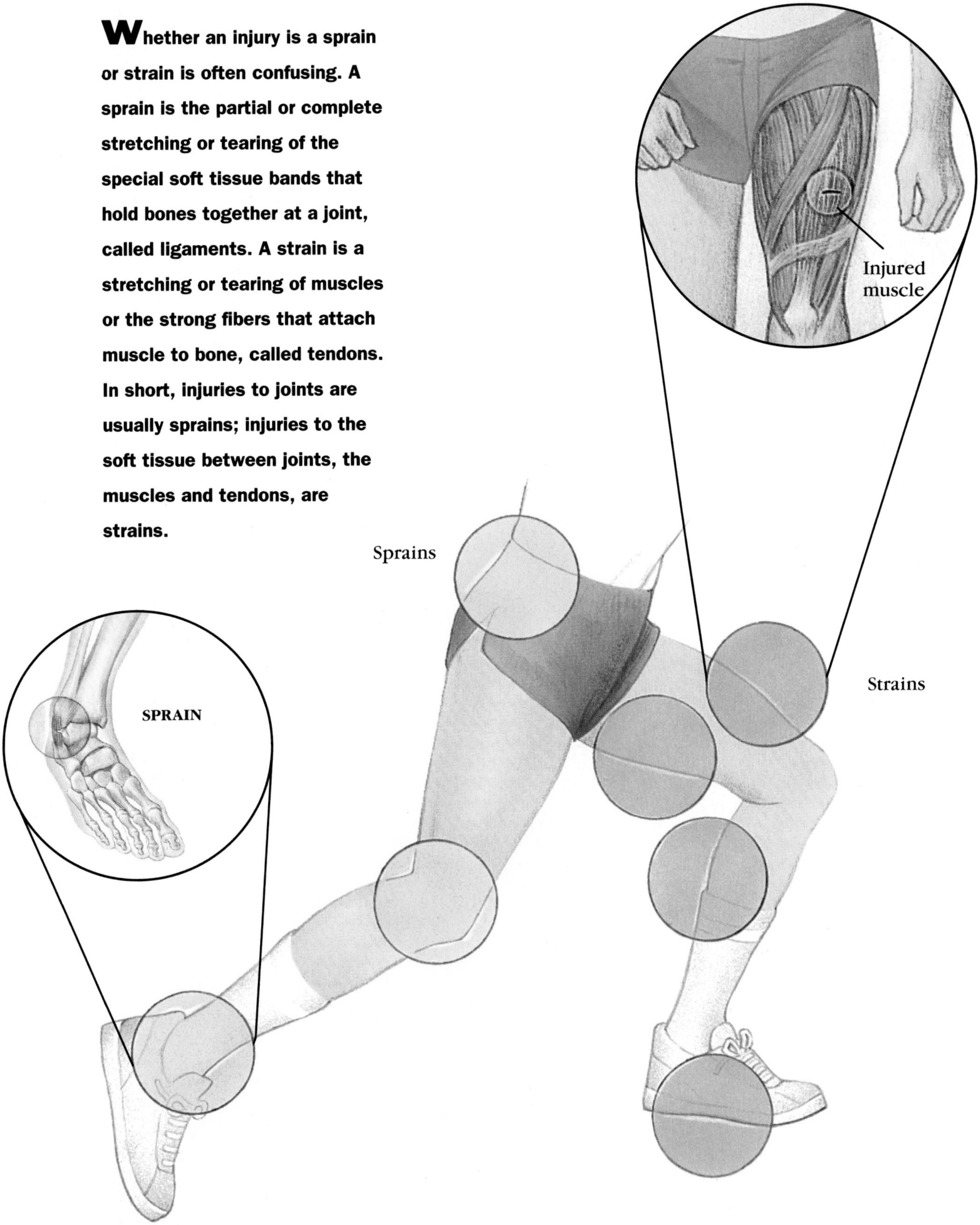

Injured muscle

Sprains

Strains

SPRAIN

IF YOU SUSPECT
A SERIOUS
MUSCLE, BONE, OR
JOINT INJURY, YOU
MUST KEEP THE
INJURED PART FROM
MOVING

A good way to tell if an area is not normal is to compare it with an un-injured part. For example, if you compare an arm you think may be fractured or dislocated with the un-injured one, you may be able to spot anything that looks strange or out of place. The victim may hear a snap or pop at the time of the injury or feel bones grating. Hands and fingers or feet and toes may feel numb or tingly.

When caring for a muscle, bone, or joint injury, always check and care for life-threatening conditions first, even if the victim is in pain. Then check for other injuries. If you find what appears to be an injury to a muscle, bone, or joint, you must decide whether to call for an ambulance.

Call at once if the victim's head, neck, or back is injured, if the victim has any problem breathing, or

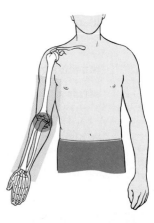

To immobilize a bone, a splint must include the joints above and below the fracture.

To immobilize a joint, a splint must include the bones above and below the injured joint.

Splinting

Splint only if the victim must be moved or transported by someone other than emergency medical personnel.

Splint only if you can do it without causing more pain and discomfort to the victim.

Splint an injury in the position you find it.

Splint the injured area and the joints above and below the injury.

Check for proper circulation before and after splinting.

if the victim is unable to move or use the injured part without pain. If you think the victim might have a head or spine injury, leave the victim lying flat.

You don't need to know what kind of injury it is to care for it. Proper care includes making the victim more comfortable. You can apply ice to control swelling and help reduce pain. Most important, minimize movement of the injured part. This can be done by helping to support it with something such as a pillow. Be careful not to move the victim in any way that causes pain.

If you are going to move or transport the victim, you must im-mobilize the injured part. One way to do this is to splint it. Splint only if you can do it without hurting the victim. Attempt to splint an injury in the position in which you find it. Splint the injured area and the joints above and below the area. Check for circulation before and after splinting to make sure the splint isn't too tight.

There are a variety of ways you can immobilize an injured body part. One method is to use the victim's body to splint an injured area. For example, you can splint an arm to the chest or an injured leg to the uninjured leg. A part of the body used as a splint is called an anatomic splint.

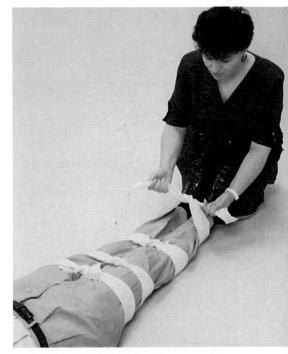

A part of the body used as a splint is called an anatomic splint. For instance, an injured leg can be splinted to the uninjured leg.

Folded blankets, towels, pillows, and a triangular bandage tied as a sling or folded as a cravat can be used as soft splints.

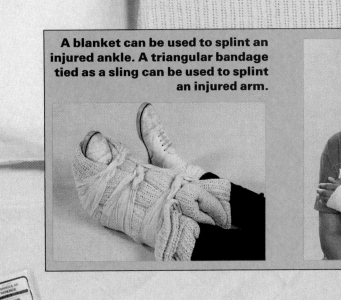

A blanket can be used to splint an injured ankle. A triangular bandage tied as a sling can be used to splint an injured arm.

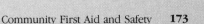

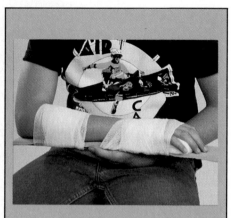

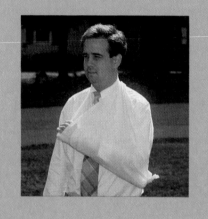

A padded rigid splint can be applied to an injured forearm.

You can make a soft splint from soft materials such as folded blankets, towels, or pillows. A soft splint can also be made from a folded triangular bandage. A sling, another kind of soft splint, is a triangular bandage tied to support an injured arm, wrist, or hand. You can also use rigid splints such as boards, folded magazines and newspapers, and metal strips to immobilize the injury.

Remember, the purpose of splinting is to keep an injured part from moving. If a victim with an injured leg is sitting or lying so that the leg is stretched out on the ground, the ground will work as a splint.

After you have splinted the injury, apply ice and raise the injured part. Keep the victim from getting chilled or overheated and be reassuring. Some injuries, such as a broken finger, don't require you to call an ambulance but still need medical attention. When transporting the victim, have someone else drive, if possible, so you can keep an eye on the victim and give any necessary care.

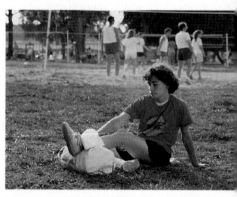

General care for all musculoskeletal injuries is similar. Remember rest, ice, and elevation.

Boards, folded newspapers, and magazines can be used as rigid splints.

Sprains and Strains

Spring is the season of flowers, trees, strains, and sprains. Almost as soon as armchair athletes come out of hibernation to become intramural heroes, emergency clinics see an increase in sprained ankles, twisted knees, and strained backs. So what do you do when you attempt the first slide of the softball season and wind up injured? Should you apply heat or apply cold?

The answer is both. First cold, then heat. It does not matter whether it is a strain or a sprain!

When a person twists an ankle or strains his or her back, the tissues underneath the skin are injured. Blood and fluids seep from the torn blood vessels and cause swelling to occur at the site of the injury. By keeping the injured area cool, you can help control internal bleeding and reduce pain. Cold causes the broken blood vessels to constrict, limiting the blood and fluid that seep out. Cold also reduces muscle spasms and numbs the nerve endings. Ice should be applied to the injury periodically for about 72 hours or until the swelling goes away.

Next, apply heat. Heat speeds up chemical reactions needed to repair the tissue. White blood cells move in to rid the body of infections, and other cells begin the repair process. This enhances proper healing of the injury. If you are unsure whether to use cold or heat on an injured area, always apply cold until you can consult your physician.

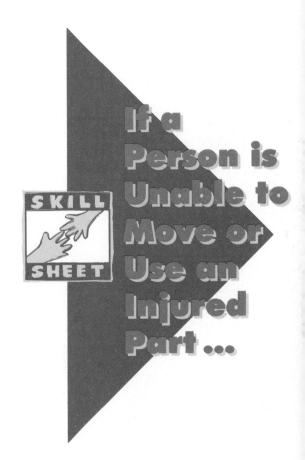

If a Person is Unable to Move or Use an Injured Part ...

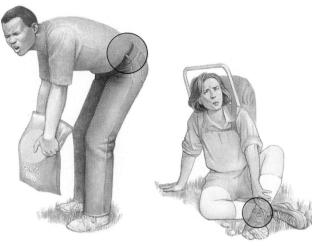

STRAIN   SPRAIN

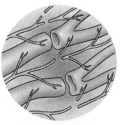

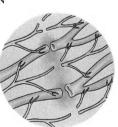

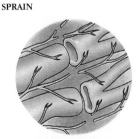

An injury causes damage to blood vessels, causing bleeding in the injured area. Injury irritates nerve endings, causing pain.

Applying ice or a cold pack constricts blood vessels, slowing bleeding that causes the injury to swell. Cold deadens nerve endings relieving pain.

Applying heat dilates blood vessels, increasing blood flow to the injured area. Nerve endings become more sensitive.

Apply an Anatomic Splint

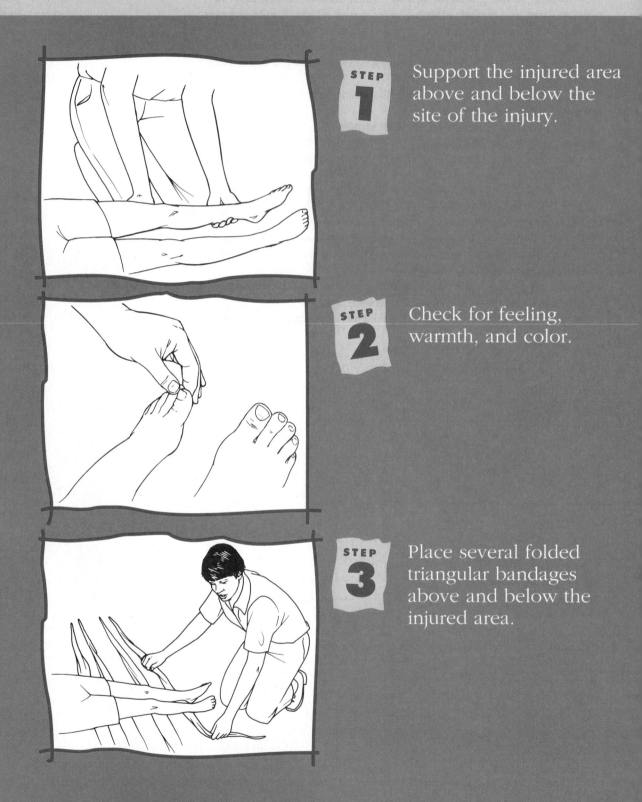

Support the injured area above and below the site of the injury.

Check for feeling, warmth, and color.

Place several folded triangular bandages above and below the injured area.

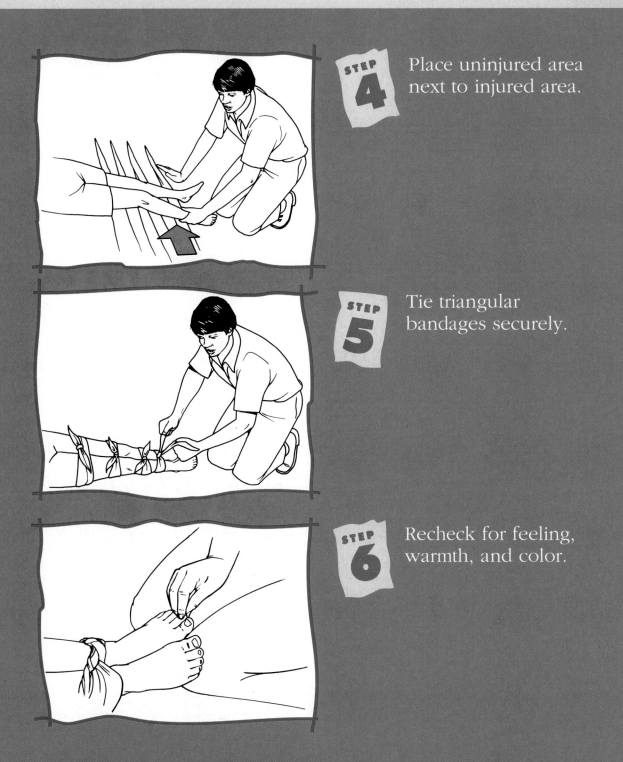

STEP 4 Place uninjured area next to injured area.

STEP 5 Tie triangular bandages securely.

STEP 6 Recheck for feeling, warmth, and color.

Apply a Soft Splint

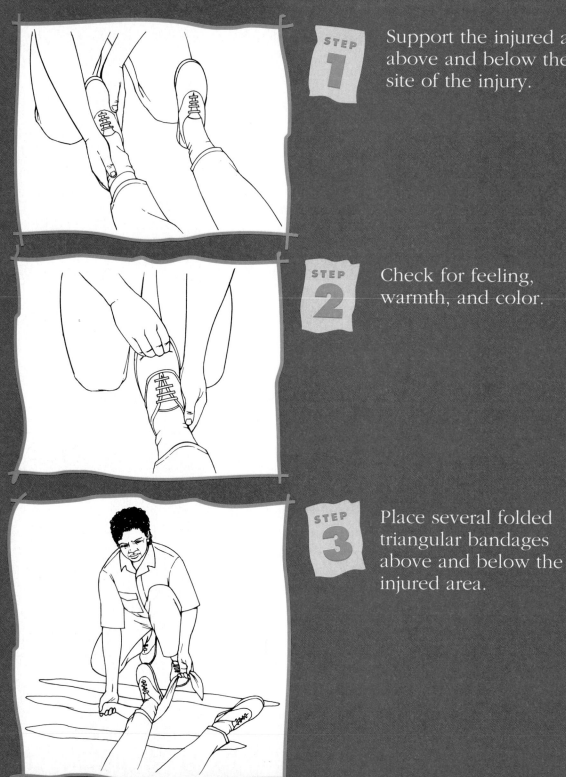

Support the injured area above and below the site of the injury.

Check for feeling, warmth, and color.

Place several folded triangular bandages above and below the injured area.

STEP **4**
Gently wrap a soft object (a folded blanket or a pillow) around the injured area.

STEP **5**
Tie triangular bandages securely.

STEP **6**
Recheck for feeling, warmth, and color.

If you are not able to check warmth and color because a sock or shoe is in place, check for feeling.

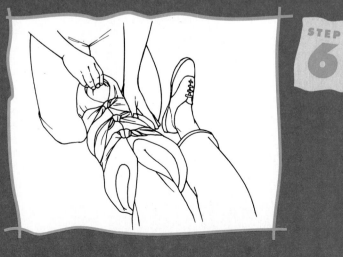

Apply a Sling

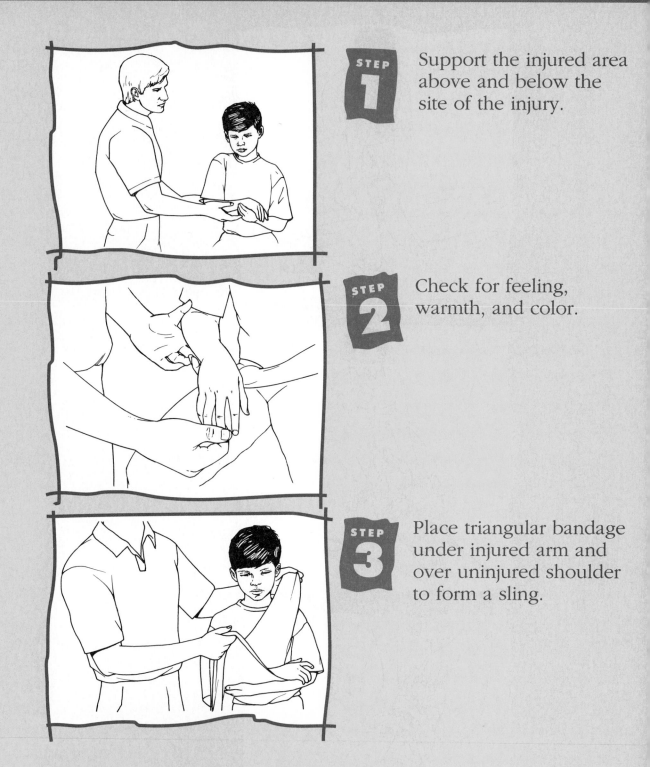

STEP 1 Support the injured area above and below the site of the injury.

STEP 2 Check for feeling, warmth, and color.

STEP 3 Place triangular bandage under injured arm and over uninjured shoulder to form a sling.

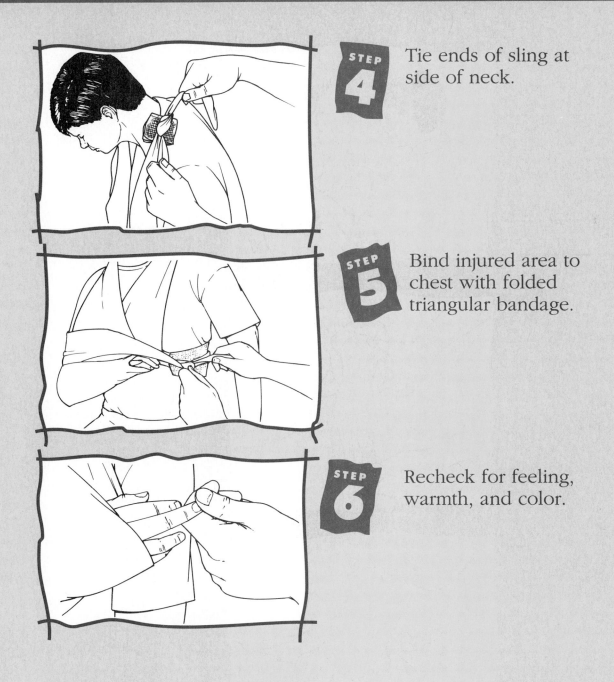

STEP 4 Tie ends of sling at side of neck.

STEP 5 Bind injured area to chest with folded triangular bandage.

STEP 6 Recheck for feeling, warmth, and color.

Apply a Rigid Splint

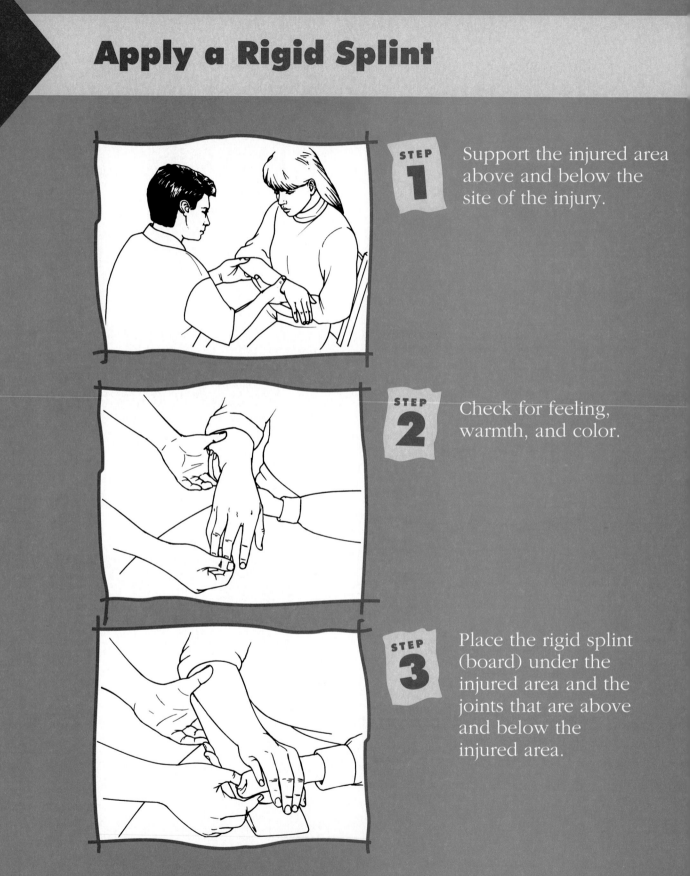

STEP 1 Support the injured area above and below the site of the injury.

STEP 2 Check for feeling, warmth, and color.

STEP 3 Place the rigid splint (board) under the injured area and the joints that are above and below the injured area.

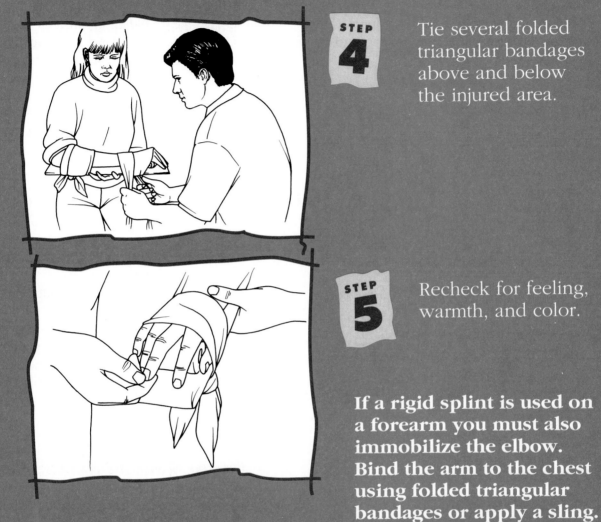

STEP 4

Tie several folded triangular bandages above and below the injured area.

STEP 5

Recheck for feeling, warmth, and color.

If a rigid splint is used on a forearm you must also immobilize the elbow. Bind the arm to the chest using folded triangular bandages or apply a sling.

SPECIAL SITUATIONS

Although head and spine injuries are only a small fraction of all injuries, they cause more than half the deaths. Each year, more than 2 million Americans suffer a head or spine injury. Most of them are males between the ages of 15 and 30. Motor vehicle crashes cause about half of all head and spine injuries. Falls, sports accidents, and acts of violence are other causes.

Injuries to the head and spine can cause paralysis, speech or memory problems, or other disabling conditions. Injuries to the head and spine can damage bone and soft tissue, including the brain and spinal cord. Since generally only x rays can show the severity of a head or spine injury, you should always care for such an injury as if it were serious.

An injury to the brain can cause bleeding inside the skull. The blood can build up and cause pressure that can cause more damage. The first and most important signal of brain injury is a change in the level of the victim's consciousness. He or she may be dizzy or confused or may become unconscious.

The spine is a strong, flexible column of small bones that supports the head and trunk. The spinal cord runs through the circular openings of the small bones, the vertebrae. The vertebrae are separated from each other by cushions of cartilage called disks. Nerves originating in the brain form branches extending to various parts of the body through openings in the vertebrae. Injuries to the spine can fracture vertebrae and tear liga-

Injuries to the head can rupture blood vessels in the brain. Pressure builds within the skull as blood accumulates, causing brain injury.

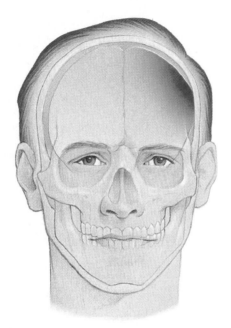

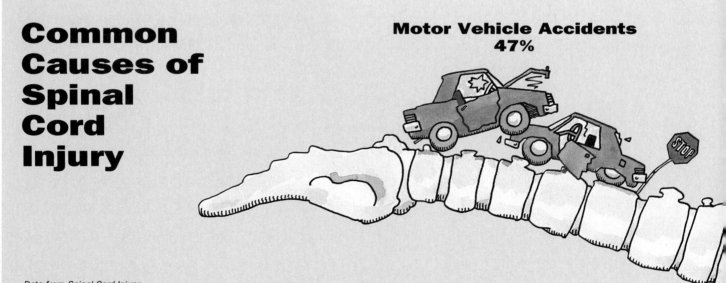

Common Causes of Spinal Cord Injury

Motor Vehicle Accidents 47%

Data from *Spinal Cord Injury; The Facts and Figures*, 1986.

WHEN TO SUSPECT HEAD AND SPINE INJURIES

A fall from a height greater than the victim's height.

Any diving mishap.

A person found unconscious for unknown reasons.

Any injury involving severe blunt force to the head or trunk, such as from a car or other vehicle.

Any injury that penetrates the head or trunk, such as a gunshot wound.

A motor vehicle crash involving a driver or passengers not wearing safety belts.

Any person thrown from a motor vehicle.

Any injury in which a victim's helmet is broken, including a motorcycle, football, or industrial helmet.

Any incident involving a lightning strike.

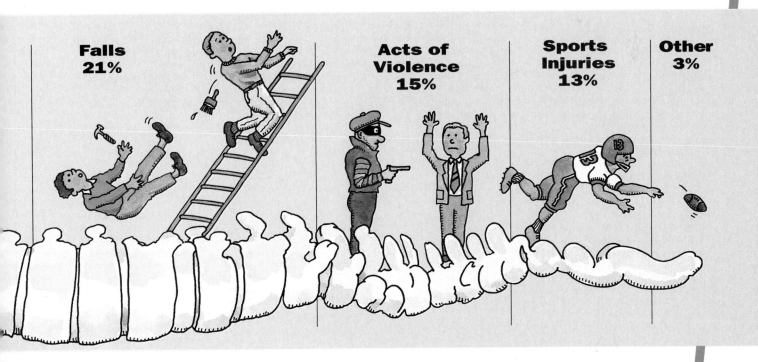

Falls 21%

Acts of Violence 15%

Sports Injuries 13%

Other 3%

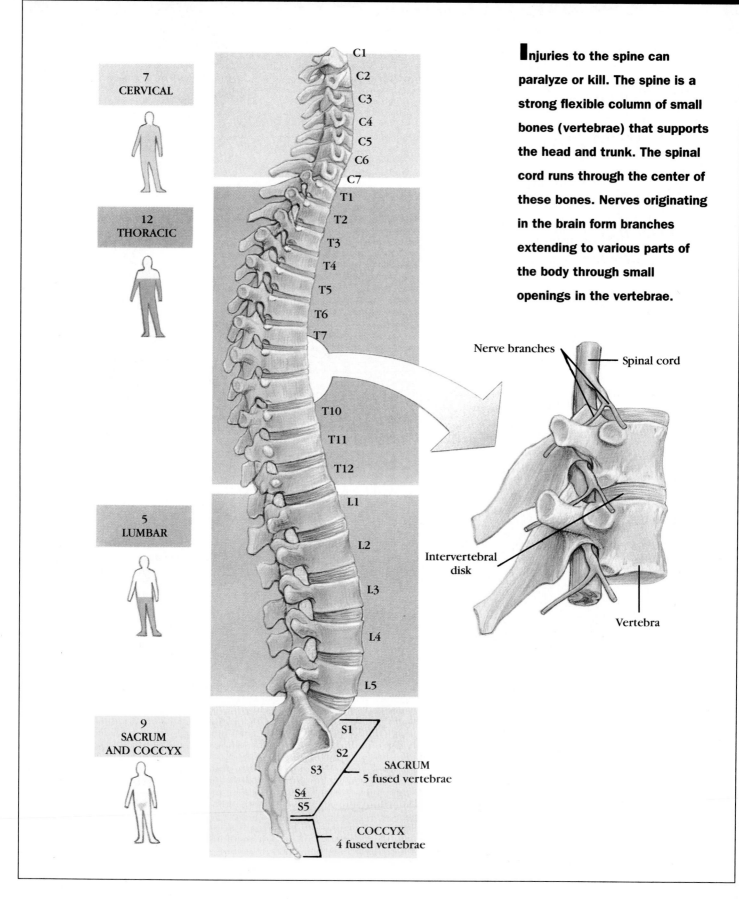

7
CERVICAL

12
THORACIC

5
LUMBAR

9
SACRUM
AND COCCYX

C1
C2
C3
C4
C5
C6
C7
T1
T2
T3
T4
T5
T6
T7
T10
T11
T12
L1
L2
L3
L4
L5
S1
S2
S3
S4
S5
SACRUM
5 fused vertebrae
COCCYX
4 fused vertebrae

Injuries to the spine can paralyze or kill. The spine is a strong flexible column of small bones (vertebrae) that supports the head and trunk. The spinal cord runs through the center of these bones. Nerves originating in the brain form branches extending to various parts of the body through small openings in the vertebrae.

Nerve branches
Spinal cord
Intervertebral disk
Vertebra

ments. In some cases the vertebrae can shift and cut or squeeze the spinal cord. This can paralyze and even kill the victim.

When you are dealing with an injured person, think whether the forces involved in the injury were great enough to cause a head or spine injury. A victim may have fallen from a height or may have struck his or her head diving. The victim might have been in a car crash and might not have been wearing a safety belt or might have been thrown from the car. The victim might have been struck by lightning. The victim's back might have been pierced by a bullet that struck the spine. Always suspect head or spine injury in a victim whose safety helmet has been broken by the injury or who is unconscious.

Besides the cause of the injury, certain signals suggest head or spine injury. They include a change in consciousness, problems with breathing and vision, inability to move a body part, ongoing headache, nausea and vomiting, and loss of balance.

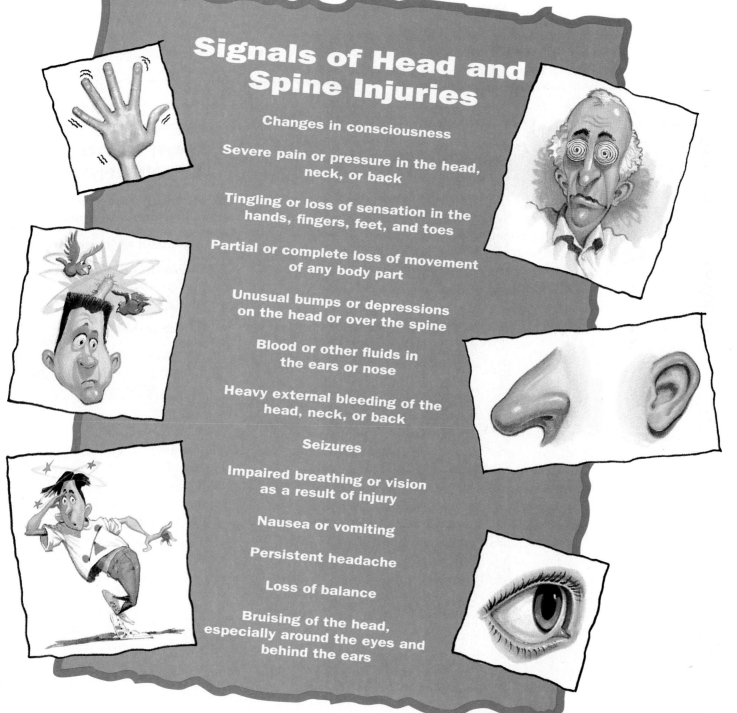

Signals of Head and Spine Injuries

Changes in consciousness

Severe pain or pressure in the head, neck, or back

Tingling or loss of sensation in the hands, fingers, feet, and toes

Partial or complete loss of movement of any body part

Unusual bumps or depressions on the head or over the spine

Blood or other fluids in the ears or nose

Heavy external bleeding of the head, neck, or back

Seizures

Impaired breathing or vision as a result of injury

Nausea or vomiting

Persistent headache

Loss of balance

Bruising of the head, especially around the eyes and behind the ears

With in-line stabilization, you support the victim's head in line with the body.

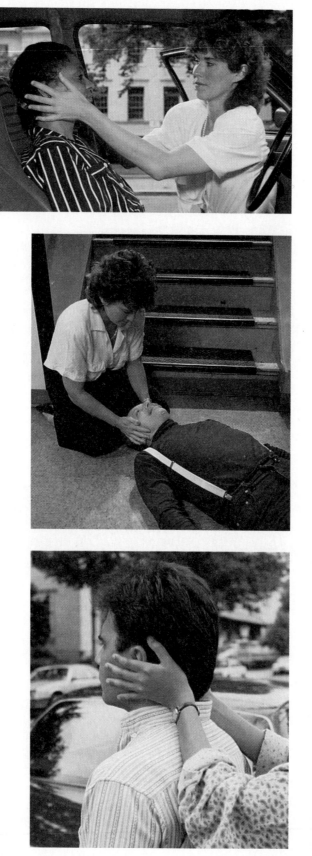

If you think a person has a head or spine injury, call for an ambulance at once. While you are waiting for the ambulance, the best care you can give is to minimize movement of the victim's head and spine. Do this by placing your hands on both sides of the victim's head. Position the head gently in line with the body and support it in that position until EMS personnel arrive. If you feel resistance as you try to do this or it hurts the victim, stop. If the head is sharply turned to one side, don't try to move it. Support the head as you found it.

GENERAL CARE FOR HEAD AND SPINE INJURIES

Minimize movement of the head and spine.

Maintain an open airway.

Check consciousness and breathing.

Control any external bleeding.

Keep the victim from getting chilled or overheated.

The victim may become confused, drowsy, or unconscious. Breathing may stop. The victim may be bleeding. If the victim is unconscious, you need to keep the airway open and check breathing. You should control any severe bleeding and keep the victim from getting chilled or overheated. Remember, if you think the victim may have a head or spine injury, call immediately for an ambulance.

Chest injuries are the second leading cause of injury deaths each year. Approximately 35 percent of all traffic deaths in the United States involve chest injuries. Injuries to the chest may also result from falls, sports mishaps, and crushing or penetrating forces.

Chest injuries range from a simple broken rib to serious life-threatening injuries. Although painful, a simple broken rib is rarely life-threatening. A victim with a broken rib will take small, shallow breaths because normal or deep breathing is painful. The victim will experience pain at the site of the injury. The victim will usually try to ease the pain by supporting the area with a hand or arm. If the injury is serious, the victim will have difficulty breathing. The victim's skin may appear flushed, pale, or bluish and he or she may cough up blood. Always consider that a person with a serious chest injury may also have a spine injury.

If you suspect injured ribs, have the victim rest in a position that will make breathing easier. Binding the

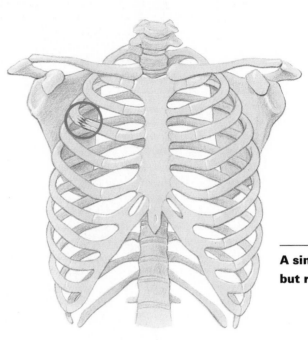

A simple rib fracture is painful but rarely life-threatening.

victim's arm to the chest on the injured side will help support the injured area and make breathing more comfortable. You can use an object, such as a pillow or folded blanket, to support and immobilize the area. If you think the injury is serious or the spine has also been injured, have the victim lie flat. Continue to watch the victim until an ambulance arrives.

The large, heavy bones of the hip are called the pelvis. Like the chest, injury to the pelvic bones can range from simple to life-threaten-ing. Because these large bones help to protect important organs inside the body, severe forces can cause heavy internal bleeding. Although a serious injury may be immediately obvious, some may develop over time.

Because an injury to the pelvis can also injure the lower spine, it is best not to move the victim. If possible, try to keep the victim lying flat. Watch for signals of internal bleeding and take steps to mini-mize shock until the ambulance arrives.

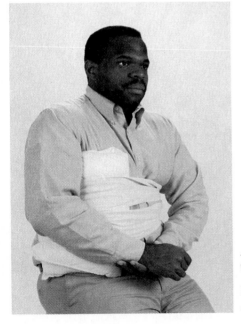

When a rib fracture occurs, use a pillow or folded blanket to support and immobilize the injured area.

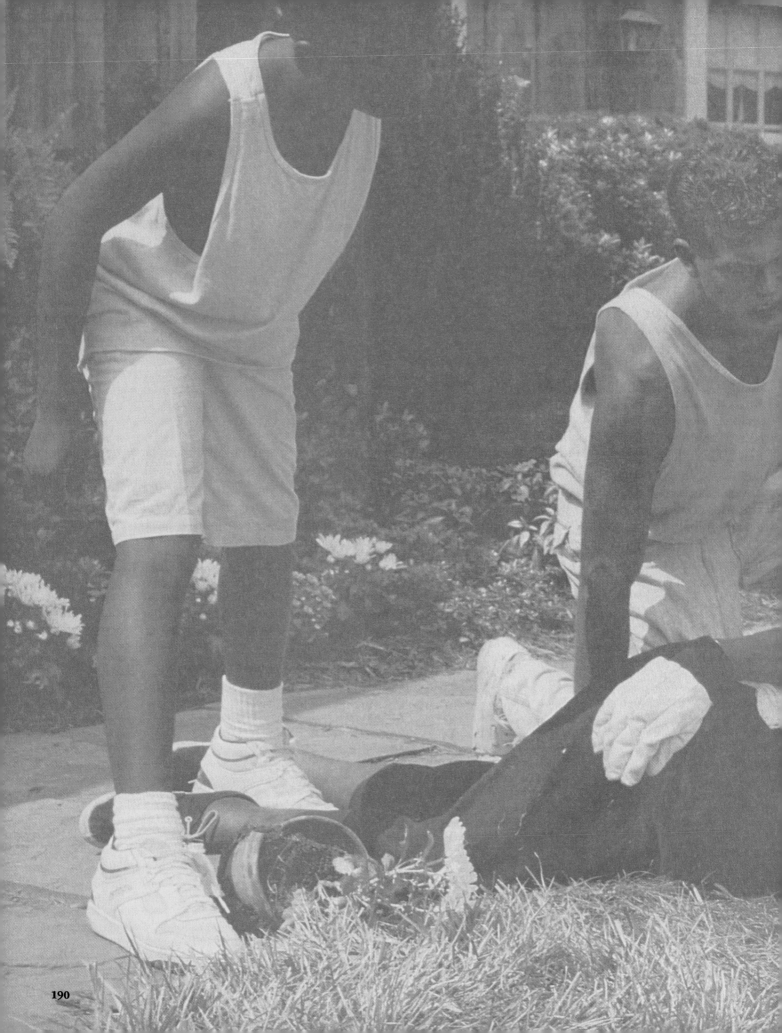

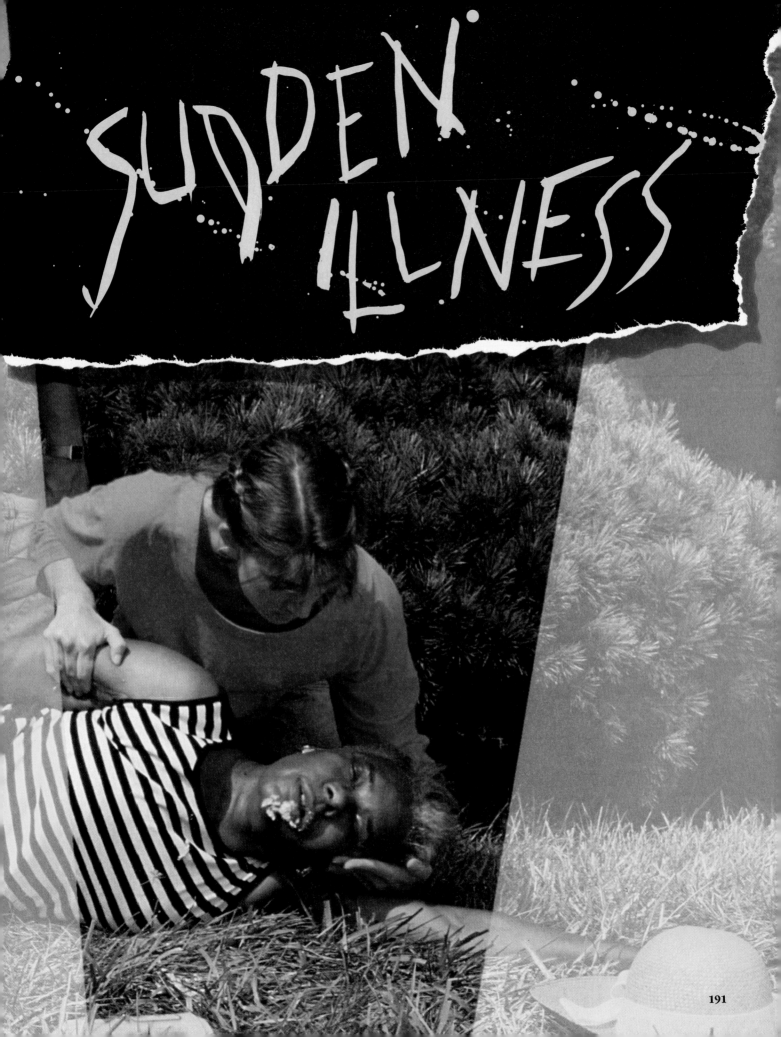

SUDDEN ILLNESS

It's usually obvious when someone is injured and needs care. The victim may be able to tell you what happened and what hurts. Checking the victim also gives you clues about what might be wrong. When someone becomes suddenly ill, however, it is not as easy to tell what is wrong. At times there are no warning signals to give clues about what is happening. At other times, the signals only confirm that something is wrong. In either case the signals of a sudden illness are often confusing. You may find it difficult to determine if the victim's condition is an emergency and whether or not to call an ambulance.

RECOGNIZING SUDDEN ILLNESS

Although there are many different types of sudden illnesses, they often have similar signals. Victims generally look ill. The signals include changes in consciousness, such as feeling light-headed or dizzy or becoming unconscious, and nausea or vomiting. The victim may have difficulty speaking or complain of numbness or paralysis. You may see changes in breathing. The victim may have trouble breathing or may not be breathing normally. The victim's skin may become pale or flushed and the victim may be sweating. The victim may be in pain or have difficulty moving.

Besides the physical signals you see, you may also be able to get some clues by looking at the victim's location and at what he or she was doing when the illness started. For example, if someone working in a hot environment suddenly becomes ill, it would make sense to

SIGNALS OF SUDDEN ILLNESS

When a person becomes suddenly ill, he or she often looks and feels sick. Common signals include:

Feeling light-headed, dizzy, confused, or weak

Changes in skin color (pale or flushed skin), sweating

Nausea or vomiting

Diarrhea

Some sudden illnesses may also include:

Changes in consciousness

Seizure

Paralysis or inability to move

Slurred speech

Difficulty seeing

Severe headache

Breathing difficulty

Persistent pressure or pain

suspect the illness is the result of the heat. If someone suddenly feels ill or is behaving strangely and is attempting to take medication, the medication may be a clue to what is wrong. For example, the person may take

IF A PERSON BECOMES SUDDENLY ILL, DON'T SECOND GUESS, CALL EMS.

medication for a heart condition, epilepsy, or diabetes.

With some sudden illnesses, you might not be sure whether to call the local emergency number for help. Sometimes the signals come and go. However, if you can't sort the problem out quickly and easily or if you have any doubts about the severity of the illness, call your local emergency number for help. It's better to be safe than sorry.

GENERAL CARE FOR SUDDEN ILLNESS

Usually you will not know the exact cause of the sudden illness, but this should not keep you from providing appropriate care. This is because you will initially care for the signals present, not for any specific condition. In the few cases

SEIZURES

When the normal workings of the brain are disrupted by injury, disease, fever, or infection, the electrical activity of the brain becomes irregular. This can cause a loss of body control known as a seizure. Seizures may be caused by extreme heat, a diabetic condition, or an injury to the brain, for example.

Seizures may be caused by an acute or chronic condition. The chronic condition is known as epilepsy. About 2 million Americans have epilepsy. Epilepsy is usually controlled with medication. Still, some people with epilepsy have seizures from time to time. Others who go a long time without a seizure may think the condition has gone away and stop taking their medication. These people may then have a seizure again.

The person may experience an aura before the seizure occurs. An aura is an unusual sensation or feeling such as a visual hallucination; a strange sound, taste, or smell; or an urgent need to get to safety. If the person recognizes the aura, he or she may have time to tell bystanders and sit down before the seizure occurs.

Seizures range from mild blackouts that others may mistake for daydreaming to sudden, uncontrolled muscular contractions (convulsions) lasting several minutes. Infants and young children are at risk for seizures brought on by high fever. These are called febrile (heat-induced) seizures.

Although it may be frightening to see someone unexpectedly having a seizure, you should remember that most seizures last only for a few minutes, and the person usually recovers without problems. Since you will not likely know the cause of the seizure, make sure someone has called the local emergency number. Care for the person until help arrives by protecting the person from injury and keeping the airway clear. If there is fluid, such as saliva, blood, or vomit, in the person's mouth, roll him or her on one side so that the fluid drains from the mouth.

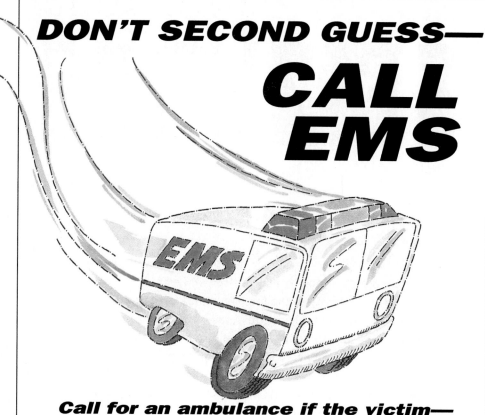

DON'T SECOND GUESS— CALL EMS

Call for an ambulance if the victim—

Is unconscious, unusually confused, or seems to be losing consciousness.

Has trouble breathing or is breathing in a strange way.

Has persistent chest pain or pressure.

Has pressure or pain in the abdomen that does not go away.

Is vomiting or passing blood.

Has seizures, severe headache, or slurred speech.

Appears to have been poisoned.

Has injuries to the head, neck, or back.

where you may know that the person has a medical condition, such as diabetes, epilepsy, or a heart condition, the care you provide may be slightly different. This care may involve helping the person take medication for his or her specific illness.

The care for sudden illnesses follows the same general guidelines as for any emergency. First, check the scene for any clues about what might be wrong. Then check the victim. Look and care for any life-threatening conditions: unconsciousness, difficulty breathing or no breathing, no pulse, severe bleeding, or severe chest pain. If the victim vomits, position the victim on his or her side. Make sure the local emergency number has been called for any life-threatening emergencies.

When providing care, always care for life-threatening conditions before those that are not life-threatening. Help the victim rest comfortably. Keep the victim from getting chilled or overheated. Reassure the victim because he or she may be anxious or frightened. Watch for changes in consciousness and breathing. If the victim is conscious, ask if he or she has any medical conditions or is taking any medication.

SPECIAL CONDITIONS

When someone suddenly loses consciousness, he or she may simply have fainted. Fainting itself is not usually harmful and the victim quickly recovers. Lower the victim to the ground or other flat surface and position him or her on the back. If possible, elevate the victim's legs 8 to 12 inches. Loosen any tight clothing, such as a tie or collar. Check to make sure the victim is breathing. Do not give the victim anything to eat or drink. If the victim vomits, place the victim on his or her side.

Since you will not be able to tell whether the fainting is a signal of a more serious condition, you should call the local emergency number.

Some illnesses that seem to come on suddenly are really caused by long-term conditions. These causes include degenerative diseases, such as heart and lung diseases. There may be a hormone imbalance, such as in diabetes. The

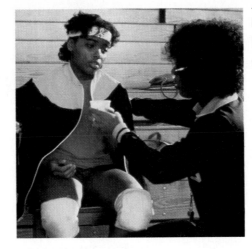

If a victim of a diabetic emergency is conscious, give him or her food or fluids containing sugar.

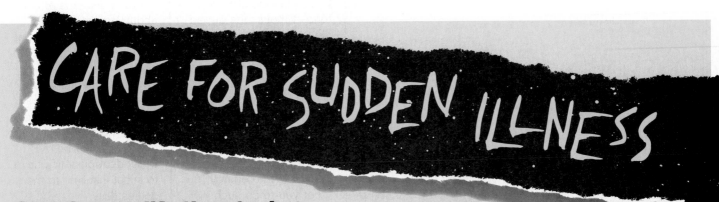

CARE FOR SUDDEN ILLNESS

Care for any life-threatening conditions first. Then:

Help the victim rest comfortably.

Keep the victim from getting chilled or overheated.

Reassure the victim.

Watch for changes in consciousness and breathing.

Do not give anything to eat or drink unless the victim is fully conscious.

If the victim:

Vomits—Place the victim on his or her side.

Faints—Position him or her on the back and elevate the legs 8 to 10 inches if you do not suspect a head or back injury.

Has a diabetic emergency—Give the victim some form of sugar.

Has a seizure—Do not hold or restrain the person or place anything between the victim's teeth. Remove any nearby objects that might cause injury. Cushion the victim's head using folded clothing or a small pillow.

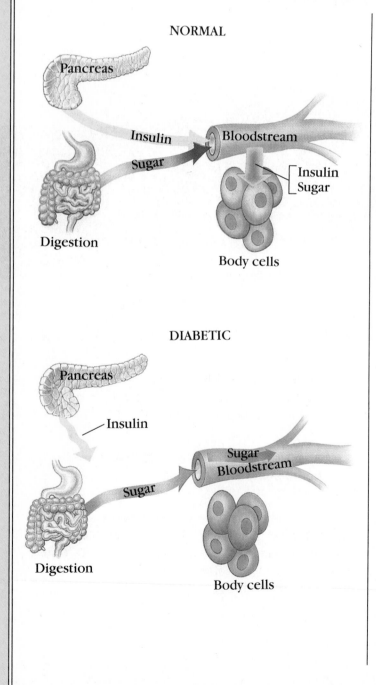

Diabetes: A Silent Killer

FYI

NORMAL

Pancreas

Insulin

Bloodstream

Sugar

Insulin
Sugar

Digestion

Body cells

DIABETIC

Pancreas

Insulin

Sugar
Bloodstream

Sugar

Digestion

Body cells

Diabetes is a leading cause of death in the United States, affecting tens of thousands of people.[1] Diabetes can lead to other medical conditions such as blindness, kidney disease, heart disease, and stroke.[2] According to the American Diabetes Association, "Diabetes is the inability of the body to properly convert sugar from food into energy."

For you to do such things as exercise, the cells in your body need sugar as a source of energy. The cells receive this energy during digestion, when the body breaks food into sugars. The sugar then becomes absorbed into the blood with the help of a hormone called insulin. Insulin is produced in the body and takes sugar into the cells. For the body to function properly, there has to be a balance of insulin and sugar in the body or the cells will starve.

When insulin is not produced or used in the proper amount, diabetes occurs. There are two major types of diabetes: Type I, insulin-dependent diabetes and Type II, noninsulin-dependent diabetes.

Type I diabetes affects about 1 million Americans.[3] This type of diabetes usually begins in childhood and is often called juvenile diabetes. This type of diabetes occurs when the body produces little or no insulin. Therefore most insulin-dependent diabetics have to inject insulin into their bodies daily.

The exact cause of juvenile diabetes is not known. Warning signs and symptoms of Type I diabetes include the following[3]:

- Increased urination
- Increased hunger and thirst
- Unexpected weight loss
- Irritability
- Weakness and fatigue

The most common type of diabetes is Type II diabetes, which affects about 90 percent of individuals with diabetes.[4] This condition is called maturity-onset diabetes and usually occurs in adults. With Type II, noninsulin-dependent diabetes, the body produces insulin but not in the necessary amounts.

According to the American Diabetes Association,

DIABETIC EMERGENCIES

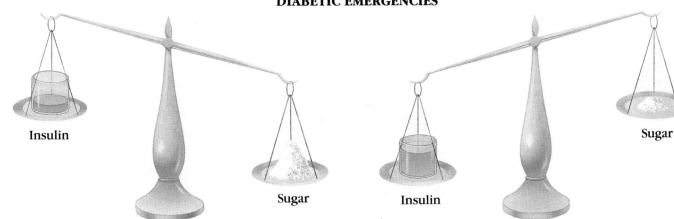

Insulin

Sugar

DIABETIC COMA (HYPERGLYCEMIA)

Insulin

Sugar

INSULIN REACTION (HYPOGLYCEMIA)

"Medical experts do not know the exact cause of Type II diabetes. They do know Type II diabetes runs in families. A person can inherit a tendency to get Type II diabetes, but it usually takes another factor, such as obesity, to bring on the disease."

Warning signs of Type II diabetes include the following[2]:

- Any symptoms of Type I diabetes
- Frequent infections
- Blurred vision
- Numbness in legs, feet, and fingers
- Cuts that are slow to heal
- Itching

It is important for all individuals with diabetes to monitor their exercise and diet. Insulin-dependent diabetics must monitor their use of insulin. If a diabetic does not control these factors, an imbalance between insulin and sugar in the body can create a diabetic emergency. Signals and symptoms of a diabetic emergency include the following:

- Changes in the level of consciousness
- Rapid breathing and pulse
- Feeling and looking ill

For more information about diabetes, contact the American Diabetes Association Information Service Center 1-800-ADA-DISC or the Juvenile Diabetes Foundation at 1-800-JDF-CURE.

REFERENCES
1. National Safety Council. *Accident Facts.* 1991.
2. American Diabetes Association. *Diabetes Facts and Figures.* Alexandria, VA: Diabetes Information Service Center, 1988, updated 12/91.
3. American Diabetes Association. *What Is Insulin-Dependent Diabetes?* Alexandria, VA: Diabetes Information Service Center, 1989.
4. American Diabetes Association. *What Is Non–Insulin-Dependent Diabetes?* Alexandria, VA: Diabetes Information Service Center, 1989.

victim could have epilepsy, a condition that causes seizures. An allergy can cause a sudden and sometimes dangerous reaction to certain substances.

People who are diabetic sometimes become ill because there is too much or too little sugar in their blood. The signals of a diabetic emergency are the same as for any other sudden illness. They require the same care. You may know the victim is a diabetic or the victim may tell you he or she is a diabetic. Often diabetics know what is wrong and will ask for something with sugar in it. They may carry some form of sugar with them in case they need it.

If the victim is conscious and can take food or fluids, give him or her sugar. Most candy, fruit juices, and nondiet soft drinks have enough sugar to be effective. You can also give table sugar, either dry or dissolved in a glass of water. If the person's problem is low sugar, the sugar will help quickly. If the problem is too much sugar, the sugar will not cause any further harm. If the person does not feel better within about 5 minutes after taking sugar, call your local emergency number.

If the person is unconscious or about to lose consciousness, do not

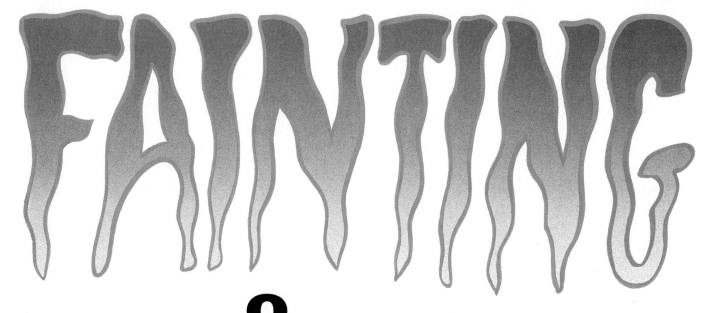

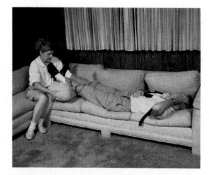

To care for fainting, place the victim on his back, elevate the feet, and loosen any restrictive clothing, such as a belt, tie, or collar.

One common signal of sudden illness is losing consciousness, such as when a person faints. Fainting is a temporary loss of consciousness. Fainting itself is not usually harmful. A person who is about to faint often becomes pale, begins to perspire, and then loses consciousness and collapses.

Fainting occurs when there is an insufficient supply of blood to the brain for a short period of time. This condition results from a widening of the blood vessels in the body which causes blood to drain away from the brain. A person who feels weak or dizzy may prevent a fainting spell by lying down or sitting with the head level with the knees.

Usually the victim of fainting recovers quickly with no lasting effects. But what appears to be a simple case of fainting may actually be a signal of a more serious condition. The victim may also be injured from falling. You should always call the local emergency number for an ambulance.

give him or her anything by mouth. Instead, call your local emergency number and care for the victim in the same way as you would care for any unconscious person. This includes making sure the person's airway is clear of vomit and checking breathing and pulse until help arrives.

Stroke is another cause of sudden illness that requires prompt medical care. A person who has had a stroke will show many of the common signals of other sudden illnesses.

Care for the person as you would for anyone else who is suddenly ill. Help the victim rest comfortably. Comfort the victim. He or she might not understand what has happened. Do not give anything to eat or drink. If the victim is unconscious or drooling or is having difficulty swallowing, place him or her on one side to help drain fluids from the mouth. Call the local emergency number immediately.

Sometimes a person who becomes suddenly ill may have a seizure. Although it may be frightening to see someone unexpectedly having a seizure, you can easily help care for the person. Remember that he or she cannot control the seizure. Do not try to stop the seizure. Do not hold or restrain the person.

Care for the seizure victim as you would for any unconscious person. To protect the seizure victim from injury, remove any nearby objects that might cause injury. Protect the victim's head by placing a thin cushion under it. Folded clothing makes an adequate cushion. If there is fluid in the victim's mouth, such as saliva, blood, or vomit, roll him or her on one side so that the fluid drains from the mouth.

Do not try to place anything between the victim's teeth. People

IF A PERSON BECOMES SUDDENLY ILL, CARE FOR ANY LIFE-THREATENING CONDITIONS FIRST.

having seizures rarely bite their tongues or cheeks with enough force to cause any significant bleeding. However, some blood may be present.

When the seizure is over, the victim usually begins to breathe normally. He or she may be drowsy and disoriented. Check to see if the victim was injured during the seizure. Be reassuring and comforting. If the seizure occurred in public, the victim may be embarrassed and self-conscious. Ask bystanders not to crowd around the victim. He or she will be tired and want to rest. Stay with the victim until he or she is fully conscious and aware of the surroundings.

If the victim is known to have occasional seizures, you do not have to call EMS immediately. The victim will usually recover from a seizure in a few minutes. However, call your local emergency number if—

• The seizure lasts more than a few minutes.

• The victim has repeated seizures.
• The victim appears to be injured.
• You are uncertain about the cause of the seizure.
• The victim is pregnant.
• You know the victim is a diabetic.
• You know the victim has not had a seizure before.
• The seizure takes place in water.
• The victim does not regain consciousness after the seizure.

Having to deal with a sudden illness can be scary, especially when you don't know what is wrong. Don't hesitate to provide care. Remember, you don't have to know the cause to help. As you can see, the signals for sudden illnesses are very similar to other conditions, and the care involves skills that you already know.

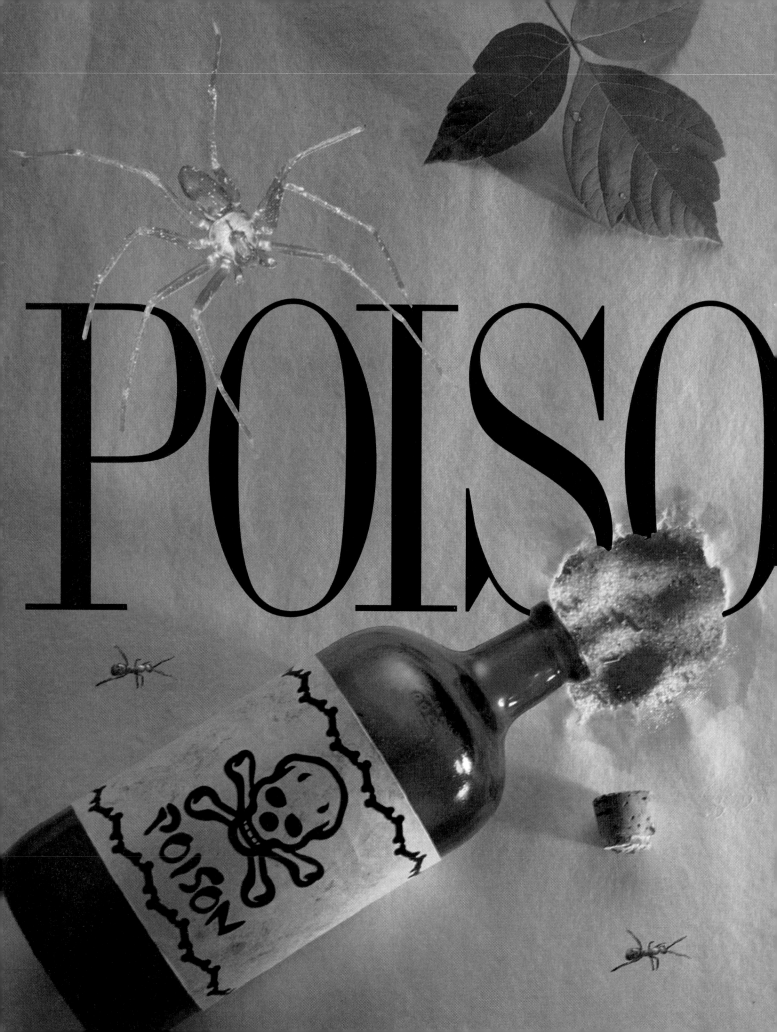

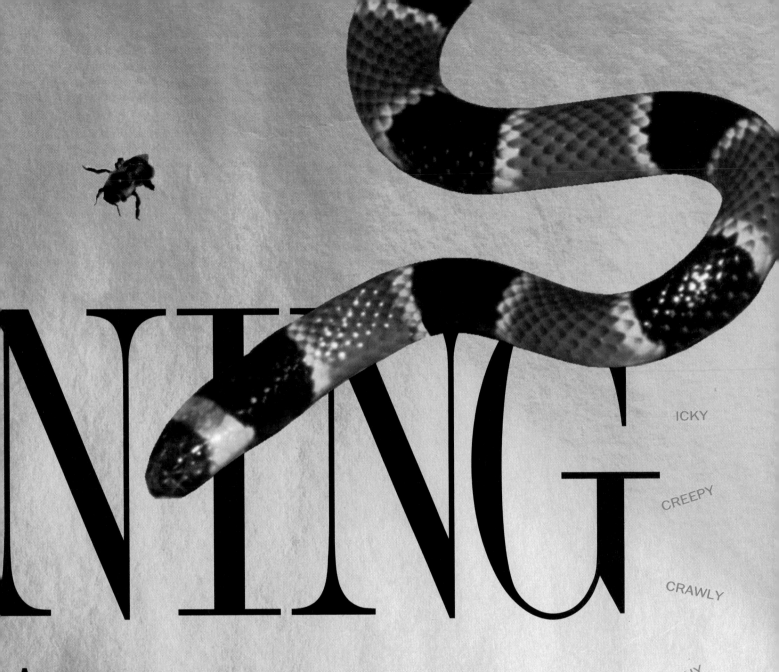

ICKY

CREEPY

CRAWLY

ITCHY

A poison is a substance that causes injury or illness if it gets into the body. Some poisons can cause death. There are four ways a person can be poisoned: by swallowing the poison, by breathing it, by absorbing it through the skin, and by having it injected into the body.

Between 1 and 2 million poisonings occur each year in the United States. More than 90 percent of all poisonings take place in the home. Most poisonings happen to children under age 5, but fewer than 5 percent of these children die. Poisoning deaths in children under age 5 have dropped in the last 30 years, but poisoning deaths among adults 18 and older have greatly increased.

The decrease in child poisonings is the result of packaging for drugs and medications that makes these substances harder for children to get into. It is also a result of preventive actions by parents and others who care for children. The increase in adult poisoning deaths is linked to an increase in suicides and increases in drug-related poisonings.

Poisons a person can swallow include foods, such as certain mushrooms and shellfish; alcohol; medications, such as aspirin; household and garden items, such as cleaning products and pesticides; and certain plants. Many substances not poisonous in small amounts are poisonous in larger amounts. Misusing and abusing certain drugs,

Watch Your Step

Annually, millions of people suffer from contact with poisonous plants whose poisons are absorbed into the body.

How many times have you been told, "Watch your step ... there's poison ivy?" Would you know what to look for? Could you identify it before you started itching? Millions of people each year suffer from contact with poisonous plants such as poison ivy, poison oak, and poison sumac.

To care for poison plant contact, immediately wash the affected area thoroughly with soap and water. If a rash or weeping sore has

eek!

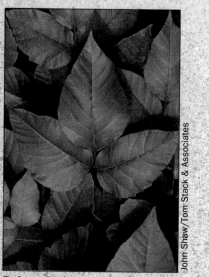
Poison Ivy

John Shaw/Tom Stack & Associates

uh oh!

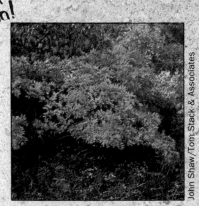
Poison Sumac

John Shaw/Tom Stack & Associates

up the sores. If the condition gets worse and affects large areas of the body or the face, see a doctor. It may be necessary to give anti-inflammatory drugs, such as corticosteroids, or other medications to relieve discomfort.

whoops!

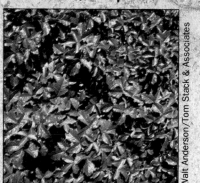
Poison Oak

Walt Anderson/Tom Stack & Associates

already begun to develop, put a paste of baking soda and water on the area several times a day to reduce the discomfort. Lotions, such as Calamine or Caladryl, may help soothe the area. Antihistamines, such as Benadryl, may also help dry

such as sleeping pills, tranquilizers, and alcohol, can also result in poisoning. Combinations of certain substances, such as drugs and alcohol, can be poisonous, although if taken by themselves they might not cause harm.

Poisoning can also result from breathing toxic fumes. Inhaled poisons may be gases, such as carbon monoxide from an engine or car exhaust; carbon dioxide from wells and sewers; and chlorine, found in many swimming pools. Inhaled poisons also include fumes from household products, such as glues, paints, and cleaners, and fumes from drugs, such as crack cocaine.

An absorbed poison enters the body through the skin. Absorbed poisons come from plants, such as poison ivy, poison oak, and poison sumac, as well as from fertilizers and pesticides used in lawn and plant care.

Injected poisons enter the body through bites or stings of insects, spiders, ticks, some marine life, snakes, and other animals, or through drugs or medications injected with a hypodermic needle.

How will you know if someone who is ill has been poisoned? Look for clues about what has happened. Try to get information from the victim or from any bystanders. If you suspect that the victim's condition is caused by some form of poisoning, call your Poison Control Center or local emergency number. Follow their direction. If the victim becomes violent or threatening, retreat to safety and wait for help to arrive.

As you check the scene, be aware of any unusual odors, flames, smoke, open or spilled containers, an open medicine cabinet, an overturned or damaged plant, or other signals of possible poisoning. The signals of poisoning include nausea, vomiting, diarrhea, chest or abdominal pain, breathing difficulty, sweating, changes in consciousness, and seizures. Other signals of poisoning are burns around the lips or tongue or on the skin. You may also suspect a poisoning based on any information you have from or about the victim.

If you suspect someone has swallowed a poison, try to find out—

• What type of poison it was.
• How much was taken.
• When it was taken.

This information can help you and others provide the most appropriate care.

Follow these general guidelines if you suspect someone has been poisoned:

• Check the scene to make sure it is safe to approach and to gather clues about what happened.
• Remove the victim from the source of the poison, if necessary.
• Check the victim's level of consciousness, breathing, and pulse.
• Care for any life-threatening conditions.
• If the victim is conscious, ask questions to get more information.
• Look for any containers and take them with you to the telephone.
• Call your Poison Control Center or local emergency number. Follow the directions of the Poison Control Center or the EMS dispatcher.

Do not give the victim anything to eat or drink unless medical professionals tell you to. If you don't know what the poison was and the victim vomits, save some of the vomit. The hospital may analyze it to identify the poison.

Just as it may be difficult to know if someone has swallowed poison, it may be difficult to tell if someone who is ill has been breathing toxic

MORE THAN 90 PERCENT OF ALL POISONINGS TAKE PLACE IN THE HOME.

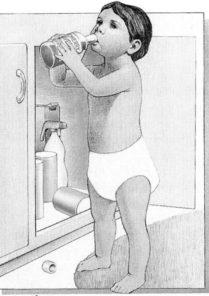

Ingestion

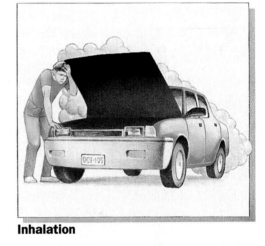

Inhalation

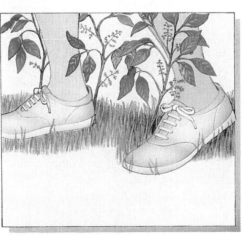

Absorption

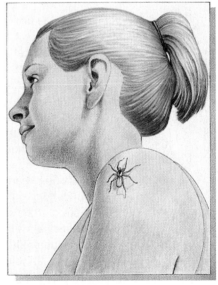

Injection

A poison can enter the body in four ways: ingestion, inhalation, absorption, and injection.

Poison Control Centers

Poison Control Centers (PCCs) help people deal with poisons. There are PCCs all over the United States. Many centers are in the emergency departments of large hospitals. The people who staff these centers have access to information about almost all poisonous substances. They will tell you how to counteract the poison.

Keep your local PCC telephone number posted by your telephone. The number will be in your telephone directory. You can also get it from your doctor, a local hospital, or your local EMS system.

Poison Control Centers answer over a million calls about poisoning each year. Many poisonings can be cared for without the help of EMS personnel, so PCCs help reduce the workload of the EMS system. If the victim is conscious, call your local or regional PCC first. The center staff will tell you what care to give and whether to call for an ambulance.

If the victim is unconscious, or if you do not know your PCC number, call your local emergency number. The dispatcher may be able to link you with the PCC. The dispatcher may also listen in to your talk with the PCC and send an ambulance if needed.

When someone has swallowed a poison, the PCC may tell you to make the victim vomit by giving syrup of ipecac. You can buy syrup of ipecac at your local drug store. It usually comes in a 30-milliliter bottle (about 2 tablespoons). Two tablespoons, followed by two glasses of water, is the normal dose for a person over 12 years of age. For children aged 1 to 12, the normal dose is 1 tablespoon followed by two glasses of water. The victim usually vomits within 20 minutes. Young children often will not take syrup of ipecac, so it may have to be given in the hospital.

There are some instances when you should not induce vomiting. This is why you should call the Poison Control Center (PCC) for advice. Do not make the victim vomit if he or she has swallowed a corrosive substance (an acid or alkali) or a petroleum product such as kerosene or gasoline. Corrosive substances burn tissues, and if vomited, can burn the esophagus, throat, and mouth.

Since vomiting removes only about half of the poison, the PCC may advise you to counteract the remaining poison with activated charcoal. You can buy it in both liquid and powder forms from drug stores. Before use, the powder should be mixed in water to form a solution with the consistency of a milk shake. For a person over 12 years of age, follow the directions on the bottle. Young children usually will not take activated charcoal, so it is given to them in the hospital.

Syrup of ipecac is used to induce vomiting in victims who have swallowed certain kinds of poisons. Activated charcoal is used to absorb swallowed poisons.

IF YOU THINK SOMEONE HAS BEEN POISONED, CALL YOUR POISON CONTROL CENTER OR LOCAL EMERGENCY NUMBER AND FOLLOW THEIR DIRECTIONS.

fumes. Toxic fumes come from a variety of sources. They may have an odor or be odor-free. A commonly inhaled poison is carbon monoxide. It is produced by gasoline-burning engines, defective cooking equipment, fires, and charcoal grills.

When someone breathes in toxic fumes, the victim's skin may may turn pale or bluish. This may mean a lack of oxygen. If it is safe for you to do so, get the victim of inhaled poison to fresh air. All victims of inhaled poison need fresh air as soon as possible.

If poisons, such as dry or wet chemicals, get on the skin, flush the affected area with large amounts of water. Call the local emergency number immediately. Keep flushing the area until EMS personnel arrive.

Dry chemicals are activated by contact with water. Continuous running water, however, will quickly flush the chemical from the skin before activating it. If running water is not available, dry chemicals, such as lime, should be brushed off. Take care not to get any in your eyes or the eyes of the victim or any bystanders.

BITES AND STINGS

Insect stings are painful, but they are rarely fatal. Some people, however, have a severe allergic reaction to an insect sting. This aller-

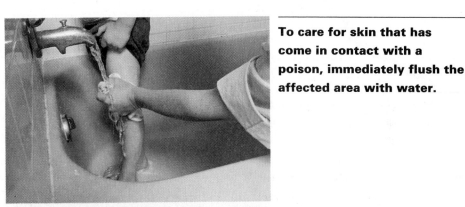

To care for skin that has come in contact with a poison, immediately flush the affected area with water.

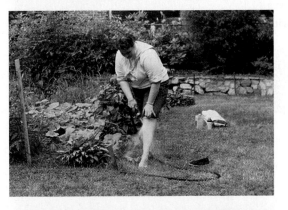

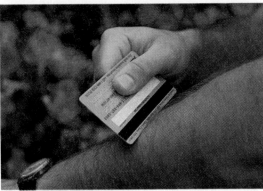

If someone is stung by an insect, remove the stinger. Scrape it away from the skin with your fingernail or a plastic card, such as a credit card.

gic reaction may result in a breathing emergency.

If someone is stung by an insect, remove the stinger. Scrape it away from the skin with your fingernail or a plastic card, such as a credit card, or use tweezers. If you use tweezers, grasp the stinger, not the venom sac. Wash the site with soap and water. Cover it to keep it clean. Apply a cold pack to the area to reduce the pain and swelling. Watch the victim for signals of an allergic reaction.

Scorpions live in dry regions of the southwestern United States and Mexico. They live under rocks, logs, and the bark of certain trees and are most active at night. Only a few species of scorpions have a sting that can cause death.

There are also only two spiders in the United States whose bite can make you seriously sick or be fatal. These are the black widow spider and the brown recluse spider. The black widow spider is black with a reddish hourglass shape on the underside of its body. The brown recluse spider is light brown with a darker brown, violin-shaped marking on the top of its body. Both spiders prefer dark, out-of-the-way places. Bites usually occur on the hands and arms of people reaching into places such as wood, rock, and brush piles or rummaging in dark garages and attics. Often, the victim

Rob Planck/Tom Stack & Associates

Black Widow

Ann Moreton/Tom Stack & Associates

Brown Recluse

Bites from the black widow spider and the brown recluse spider can make you sick or be fatal. Because both spiders prefer dark, out-of-the-way places, the victim may not know that he or she has been bitten until he or she starts to feel ill or notices a bite mark or swelling.

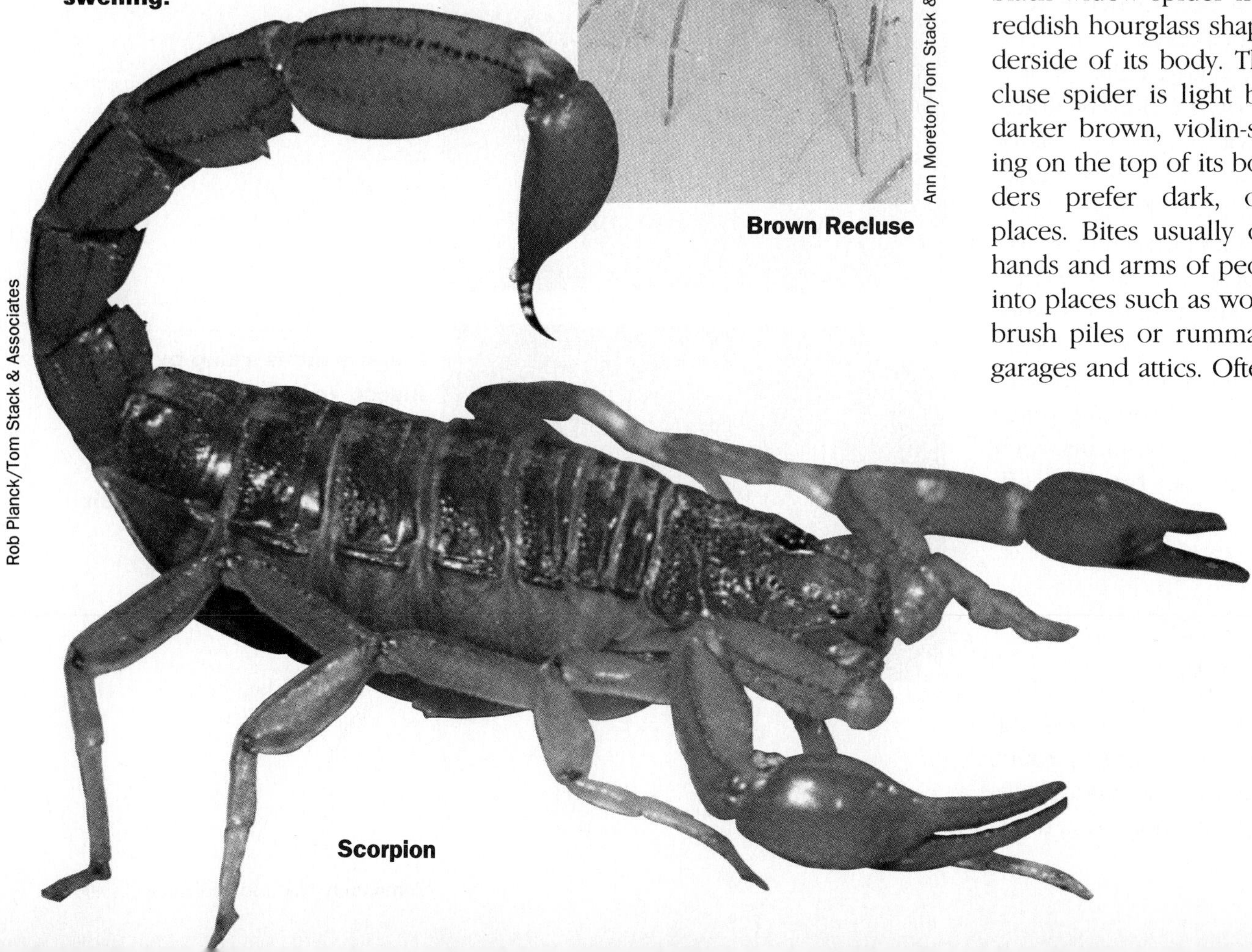

Rob Planck/Tom Stack & Associates

Scorpion

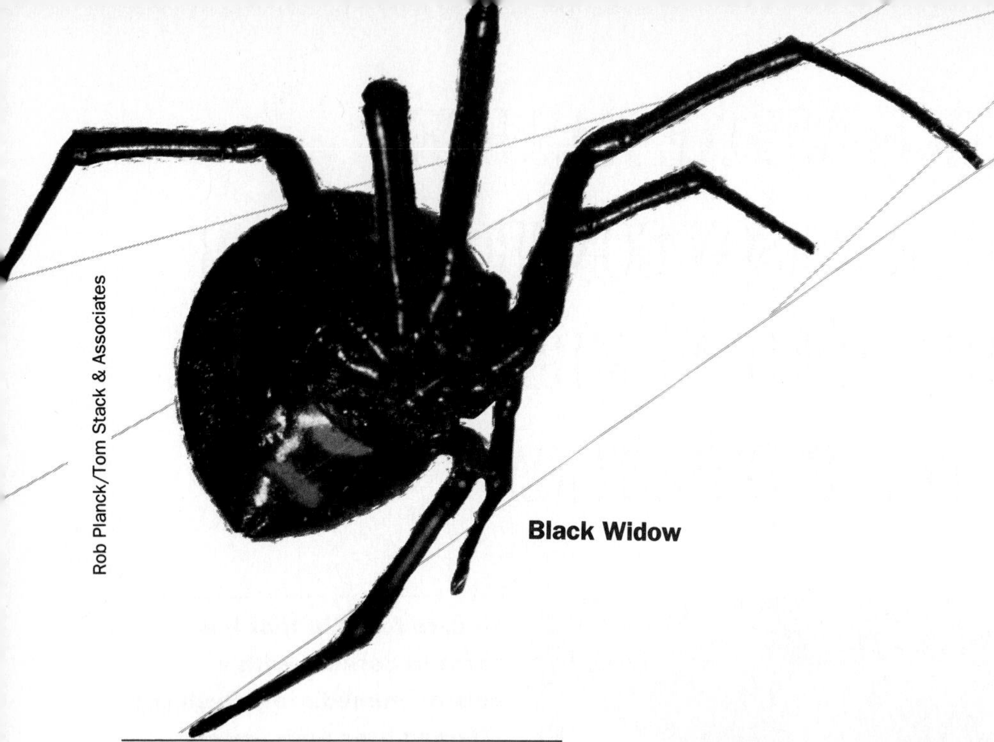

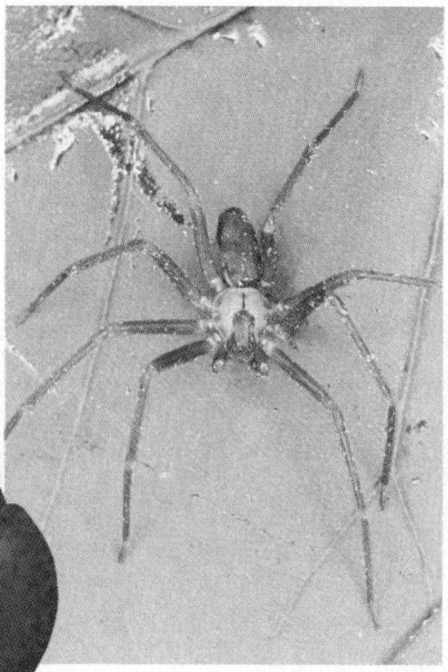

The bites of only a few species of scorpions found in the United State can be fatal.

Lyme Disease

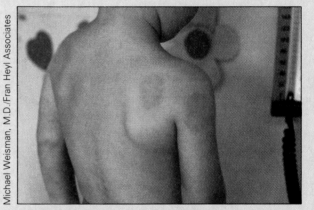

Lyme disease is an illness that people get from the bite of an infected tick. Lyme disease is affecting a growing number of people in the United States. It has occurred in more than 40 states. Everyone should take precautions to protect against it.

Not all ticks carry Lyme disease. Lyme disease is spread mainly by a type of tick that commonly attaches itself to field mice and deer. It is sometimes called a deer tick. This tick is found around beaches and in wooded and grassy areas. Like all ticks, it attaches itself to any warm-blooded animal that brushes by it, including humans. A deer tick can attach to you without your knowledge. Many people who develop Lyme disease cannot recall having been bitten.

Deer ticks are very tiny and difficult to see. They are much smaller than the common dog tick or wood tick. They can be as small as a poppy seed or the head of a pin. Adult deer ticks are only as large as a grape seed.

You can get Lyme disease from the bite of an infected tick at any time of the year. However, in northern states, the risk is greatest between May and late August, when ticks are most active and people spend more time outdoors.

The first signal of infection may appear a few days or a few weeks after a tick bite. Typically, a rash starts as a small red area at the site of the bite. It may spread up to 7 inches across. In fair-skinned people the center is lighter in color and the outer edges are red and raised. This sometimes gives the rash a bull's-eye appearance. In dark-skinned people the area may look black and blue, like a bruise.

Other signals of Lyme disease include fever, headache, weakness, and joint and muscle pain similar to the pain of "flu." These signals might develop slowly and might not occur at the same time as a rash. In fact, you can have Lyme disease without developing a rash.

Lyme disease can get worse if not treated. In its advanced stages, it may cause arthritis, numbness, memory loss, problems in seeing or hearing, high fever, and stiff neck. Some of these signals could indicate problems with the brain or nervous system. An irregular or rapid heartbeat could indicate heart problems.

If you find a tick, remove it by pulling steadily and firmly. Grasp the tick with fine-tipped tweezers, as close to the skin as possible, and pull slowly. If you do not have tweezers, use a glove, plastic wrap, or a piece of paper to protect your fingers. If you use your bare fingers, wash your hands immediately. Do not try to burn a tick off with a hot match or a burning cigarette. Do not use other home remedies, like coating the tick with Vaseline or nail polish or pricking it with a pin.

Once the tick is removed, wash the area immediately with soap and water. If an antiseptic or antibiotic ointment is available, apply it to prevent wound infection. Observe the site periodically thereafter.

If you cannot remove the tick, or if parts of the tick stay in your skin, obtain medical care. If a rash or flu-like symptoms develop, seek medical help. A physician will usually use antibiotics to treat Lyme disease. Antibiotics work best and most quickly when taken early. If you suspect Lyme disease, do not delay seeking treatment. Treatment is slower and less effective in advanced stages.

More information on Lyme disease may be available from your local or state health department.

Michael Weisman, M.D./Fran Heyl Associates

A person with Lyme disease may develop a rash.

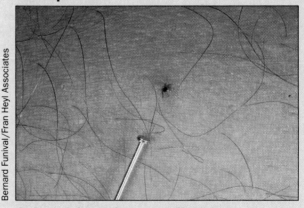

Bernard Funival/Fran Heyl Associates

A deer tick can be as small as the head of a pin.

will not know that he or she has been bitten until he or she starts to feel ill or notices a bite mark or swelling.

Signals of spider bites and scorpion stings also are similar to those of other sudden illnesses. However, if the person knows he or she has been bitten or stung, this might help identify the cause of the problem. The signals include nausea and vomiting, difficulty breathing or swallowing, sweating and salivating much more than normal, severe pain in the sting or bite area, a mark indicating a possible bite or sting, and swelling of the area.

If someone has been stung by a scorpion or bitten by a spider he or she thinks is a black widow or brown recluse, wash the wound, apply a cold pack to the site, and get medical help immediately. Antivenins are available for black widow bites and for scorpion stings. Antivenin is medication that blocks the effects of the poison.

The stings of some forms of marine life are not only painful but can also make you sick. The side effects include allergic reactions that can cause breathing and heart problems, as well as paralysis. Al-

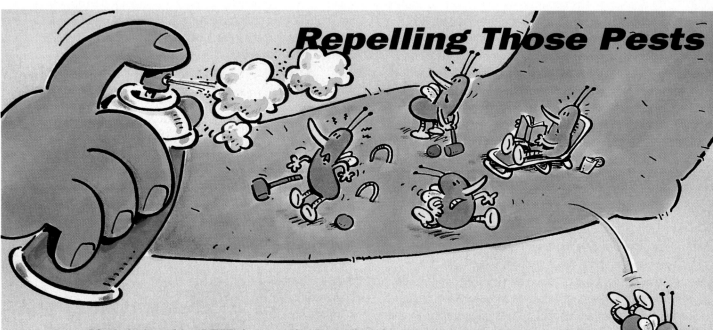

Repelling Those Pests

Diethyltoluamide (DEET) is an active ingredient in many substances called repellents, which are effective against ticks and other insects. Repellents containing DEET can be applied on exposed areas of skin and clothing. However, repellents containing permethrin, another common repellent, should be used only on clothing.

If you use a repellent, follow these general rules:

- Keep all repellents out of the reach of children.

- To apply repellent to the face, first spray it on your hands and then apply it from your hands to your face. Avoid sensitive areas, such as the lips and the eyes.

- Never use repellents on an open wound or irritated skin.

- Use repellents sparingly. One application will last 4 to 8 hours. Heavier or more frequent

applications will not increase effectiveness.

- Wash treated skin with soap and water and remove treated clothing after you come indoors.

- If you suspect you are having a reaction to a repellent, wash the treated skin immediately and call your physician.

- Never spray repellents containing permethrin on the skin.

- Never put repellents on children's hands. They may put them in their eyes or mouth.

ways remove the person from the water as soon as possible. Call 9-1-1 if the victim doesn't know what stung him or her, has a history of allergic reactions to marine life stings, is stung on the face or neck, or starts to have difficulty breathing.

If you know the sting is from a jellyfish, sea anemone, or Portugese man-of-war, soak the injured part in vinegar as soon as possible. Vinegar works best to offset the toxin, but rubbing alcohol or baking soda may also be used. Do not rub the wound or apply fresh water or ammonia because this increases pain. Meat tenderizer is no longer recommended.

If you know the sting is from a sting ray, sea urchin, or spiny fish, flush the wound with tap water. Ocean water may also be used. Immobilize the injured part, usually the foot, and soak the affected area

The painful sting of some marine animals can cause serious problems.

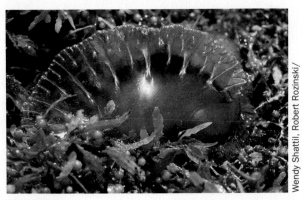

Man-o-War

Wendy Shattil, Robert Rozinski/ Tom Stack & Associates

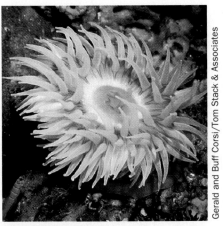

Sea Anemone

Gerald and Buff Corsi/Tom Stack & Associates

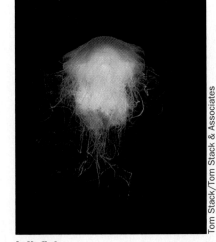

Jellyfish

Tom Stack/Tom Stack & Associates

Sting Ray

Denise Tackett/Tom Stack & Associates

Caring for Bites and Stings

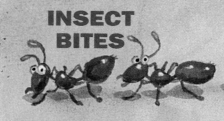

INSECT BITES

Signals

Stinger may be present

Pain

Swelling

Possible allergic reaction

Care

Remove stinger — scrape it away or use tweezers.

Wash wound.

Cover.

Apply a cold pack.

Watch for signals of allergic reaction.

SPIDER BITE / SCORPION STING

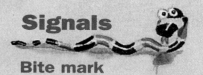

Signals

Bite mark

Swelling

Pain

Nausea and vomiting

Difficulty breathing or swallowing

Care

Wash wound.

Apply a cold pack.

Get medical care to receive antivenin.

Call local emergency number, if necessary.

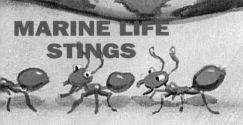

MARINE LIFE STINGS

Signals

Possible marks

Pain

Swelling

Possible allergic reaction

Care

If jellyfish—soak area in vinegar.

If sting ray—soak area in nonscalding hot water until pain goes away. Clean and bandage wound.

Call local emergency number if necessary.

SNAKE BITES

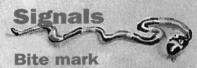

Signals

Bite mark

Pain

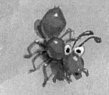

Care

Wash wound.

Keep bitten part still, and lower than the heart.

Call local emergency number.

ANIMAL BITES

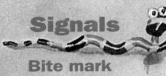

Signals

Bite mark

Bleeding

Care

If bleeding is minor—wash wound.

Control bleeding.

Apply antibiotic ointment.

Cover.

Get medical attention if wound bleeds severely or if you suspect animal has rabies.

Call local emergency number or contact animal control personnel.

SNAKEBITES KILL VERY FEW PEOPLE IN THE UNITED STATES... MOST SNAKEBITES OCCUR NEAR THE HOME, NOT IN THE WILD.

in nonscalding hot water (as hot as the person can stand) for about 30 minutes or until the pain goes away. If hot water is not available, packing the area in hot sand may have a similar effect if the sand is hot enough. Then carefully clean the wound and apply a bandage. Watch for signs of infection and check with a health care provider to determine if a tetanus shot is needed.

Snakebites kill very few people in the United States. Of the 8,000 people bitten annually in the United States, fewer than 12 die. Most snake bites occur near the home, not in the wild. Rattlesnakes account for most snakebites and nearly all deaths from snakebites. Most deaths occur because the victim has an allergic reaction, is in poor health, or because too much time passes before he or she receives medical care.

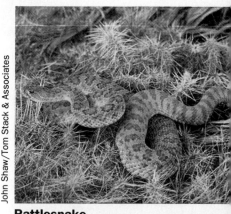

John Shaw/Tom Stack & Associates

Rattlesnake

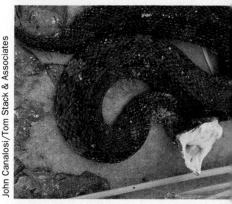

John Canalosi/Tom Stack & Associates

Water Moccasin

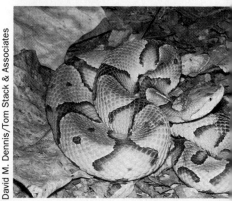

David M. Dennis/Tom Stack & Associates

Copperhead

There are four kinds of poisonous snakes found in the United States.

Coral Snake

You hear all sorts of care recommended for snakebites. To care for someone bitten by a snake, wash the wound and immobilize the injured area, keeping it lower than the heart, if possible. Call the local emergency number. Do not apply ice to a snakebite. Do not cut the wound. Do not apply a tourniquet. Do not use electric shock. If necessary, carry a victim who must be taken to a medical facility or have him or her walk slowly.

If you know the victim can't get professional medical care within 30 minutes, consider suctioning the wound using a snakebite kit, if one is available. People at risk of snakebites in the wild (away from medical care) should carry a snakebite kit and know how to use its contents.

The bite of a domestic or wild animal can cause infection and soft tissue injury. The most serious possible result is rabies. Rabies is transmitted through the saliva of diseased animals, such as skunks, bats, raccoons, cats, dogs, cattle, and foxes.

Animals with rabies may act strangely. For example, animals usually active at night, such as raccoons, may be active in the daytime. A wild animal that usually tries to avoid people might not run from you. Rabid animals may drool, appear partially paralyzed, or act irritable, mean, or strangely quiet. Do not pet or feed wild animals, and do not touch the body of a dead animal.

If not treated, rabies is fatal. Anyone bitten by an animal that might have rabies must get medical attention. To prevent rabies, the victim receives a series of vaccine injections to build up immunity that will help fight the disease.

If someone is bitten by an animal, try to get him or her away from the animal without putting yourself in danger. Do not try to stop, hold, or catch the animal. If the wound is minor, wash it with soap and water. Then control any bleeding and apply an antibiotic ointment and a dressing. Get medical attention if you suspect the animal might have rabies. Watch for signals of infection.

If the wound is bleeding seriously, control the bleeding first. Do not clean the wound. Get medical attention. The wound will be properly cleaned at a medical facility.

If possible, try to remember what the animal looked liked and the area in which you last saw it. Call your local emergency number. The dispatcher will get the proper authorities, such as animal control, to the scene.

ANYONE BITTEN BY AN ANIMAL THAT MIGHT HAVE RABIES MUST GET MEDICAL ATTENTION.

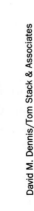

David M. Dennis/Tom Stack & Associates

MOST POISONINGS CAN BE PREVENTED.

PREVENTING POISONING

Poisonings can be prevented. This is a simple idea, but often people are not careful enough. Use common sense when handling substances that could be harmful, such as chemicals and cleaners. Use them in a well-ventilated area. Wear protective clothing, such as gloves and a face mask.

Use common sense with your own medications. Read the product information and use only as directed. Ask your doctor or pharmacist about the intended effects, side effects, and possible interactions with other medications you are taking. Never use another person's prescribed medications; what is right for one person is seldom right for another. Always keep medications in the containers they came in and make sure the container is well-marked. Destroy all out-of-date medications. Over time they can become less effective and even toxic.

HOW TO PREVENT POISONING

A child can get into trouble in just a moment. Childen are curious and can get into things in ways you might not think possible. Almost all child poisonings reported occurred when the child was being watched by a parent or guardian. Many substances found in or around the house are poisonous. Children are especially likely to be poisoned because they tend to put everything into their mouths.

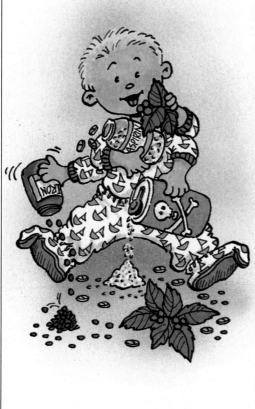

Follow these guidelines to guard against poisoning emergencies:

Children should always be closely supervised by a responsible person.

Keep all medications and household products locked away, well out of the reach of children.

Install special clamps to keep children from opening cabinets.

Consider all household or drugstore products to be potentially harmful.

Use childproof safety caps on containers of medication and other potentially dangerous products.

Never call medicine "candy" to get a child to take it, even if it has a pleasant candy flavor.

Read the label.

Keep products in their original containers with the labels in place.

Use poison symbols to identify dangerous substances, and teach children what the symbols mean.

Dispose of outdated products as recommended.

Use chemicals only in well-ventilated areas.

During work or recreation that may put you in contact with a poisonous substance, set a good example. Wear proper protective clothing, such as gloves or a mask.

How to BEAT those little critters ...

You can prevent bites and stings from insects, spiders, ticks, or snakes by following these guidelines when you are in wooded or grassy areas.

Wear long-sleeved shirts and long pants.

Tuck your pant legs into your socks or boots.

Tuck your shirt into your pants.

Wear light-colored clothing to make it easier to see tiny insects or ticks.

Use a rubber band or tape to hold pants against socks, so that nothing can get under clothing.

When hiking in woods and fields, stay in the middle of trails. Avoid underbrush and tall grass.

If you are outdoors for a long time, check yourself several times during the day. Especially check in hairy areas of the body like the back of the neck and the scalp line.

Avoid walking in areas known to be populated with snakes.

If you encounter a snake, look around, there may be others. Turn around and walk away on the same path you came on.

Inspect yourself carefully for insects or ticks after being outdoors or have someone else do it.

Wear sturdy hiking boots.

If you have pets that go outdoors, spray them with repellent made for your type of pet. Apply the repellent according to the label, and check your pet for ticks often.

If you will be in a grassy or wooded area for a long time, or if you know the area is highly infested with insects or ticks, you may want to use a repellent. (Follow the directions carefully.)

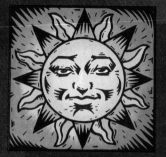

BATTLING THE

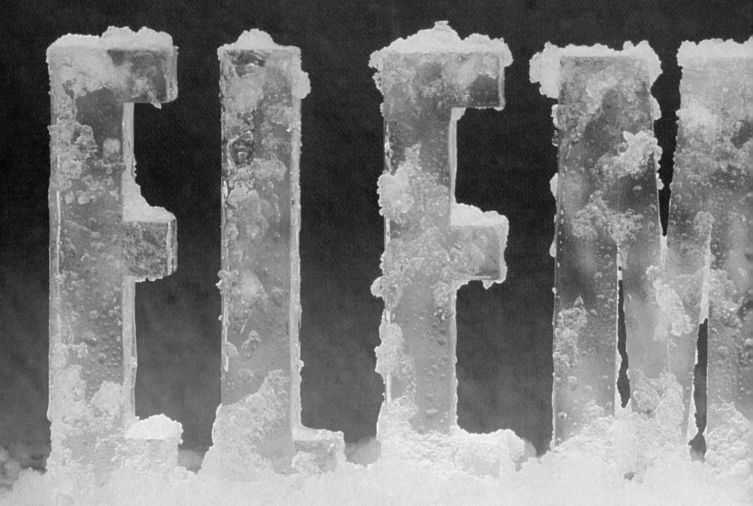

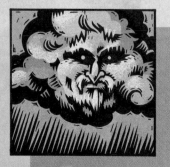

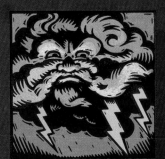

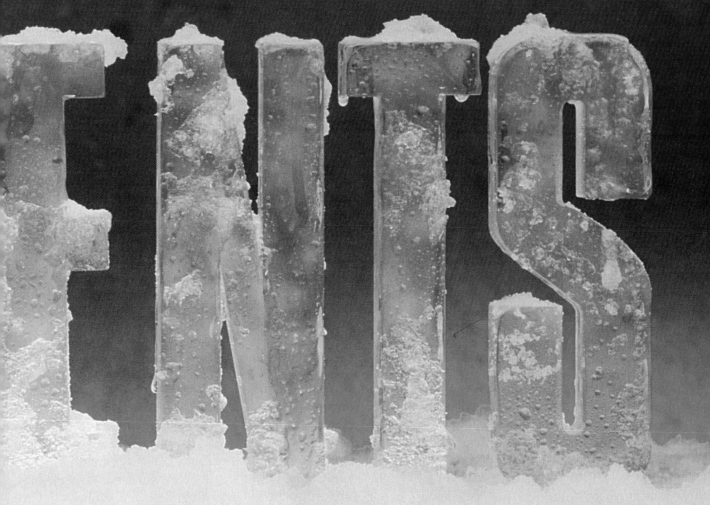
ENTS

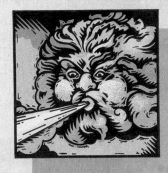

Exposure to extreme heat or cold may make a person seriously ill. The likelihood of illness also depends on factors such as physical activity, clothing, wind, humidity, working and living conditions, and a person's age and state of health.

Temperature, humidity, and wind are the three main factors affecting body temperature.

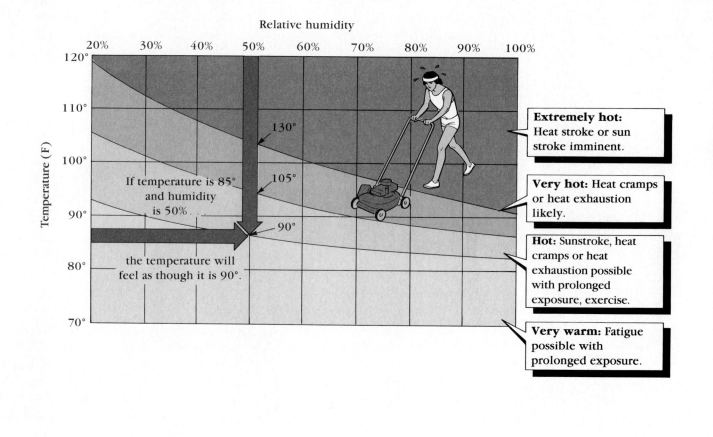

Once the signals of a heat- or cold-related illness begin to appear, the victim's condition can quickly get worse. A heat- or cold-related illness can result in death. If you see any of the signals of sudden illness and the victim has been exposed to extremes of heat or cold, suspect a heat- or cold-related illness.

People at risk for heat- or cold-related illnesses include those who work or exercise outdoors, elderly people, young children, and people with health problems. Also at risk are those who have had a heat- or cold-related illness in the past, those with medical conditions that cause poor blood circulation, and those who take medications to get rid of water from the body (diuretics).

People usually try to get out of extreme heat or cold before they begin to feel ill. However, some people do not or cannot. Athletes and those who work outdoors often keep working even after they begin to feel ill. Those living in poorly ventilated or poorly insulated buildings or with poor heating or cooling systems are at increased risk of heat or cold emergencies. Many times, they might not even recognize that they are in danger of becoming ill.

Heat-Related Illness

Heat cramps, heat exhaustion, and heat stroke are conditions caused by overexposure to heat. Heat cramps are the least severe, and often are the first signals that the body is having trouble with the heat. Heat cramps are painful muscle spasms. They usually occur in the legs and abdomen. Think of them as a warning of a possible heat-related emergency.

To care for heat cramps, have the victim rest in a cool place. Give cool water or a commercial sports drink. Usually, rest and fluids are all the person needs to recover. Lightly stretch the muscle and gently massage the area. The victim should not take salt tablets or salt water. They can make the situation worse.

When the cramps stop, the person can usually start activity again if there are no other signals of illness. He or she should keep drinking plenty of fluids. Watch the victim

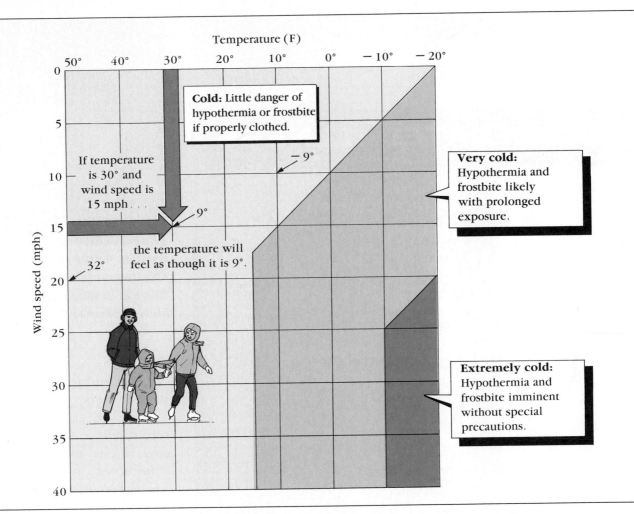

Temperature (F)

| 50° | 40° | 30° | 20° | 10° | 0° | − 10° | − 20° |

Cold: Little danger of hypothermia or frostbite if properly clothed.

If temperature is 30° and wind speed is 15 mph . . .

the temperature will feel as though it is 9°.

− 9°

9°

32°

Very cold: Hypothermia and frostbite likely with prolonged exposure.

Extremely cold: Hypothermia and frostbite imminent without special precautions.

Wind speed (mph)

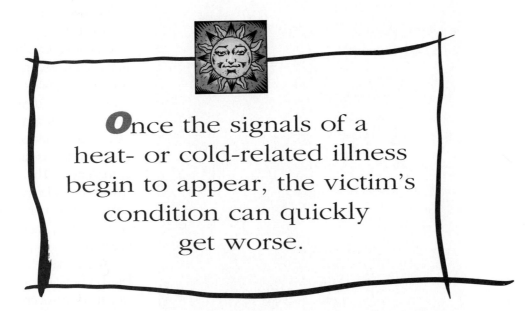

Once the signals of a heat- or cold-related illness begin to appear, the victim's condition can quickly get worse.

Caring For

HEAT-RELATED ILLNESS

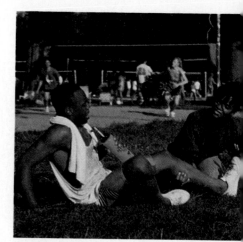

Resting, lightly stretching the affected muscle, and replenishing fluids is usually enough for the body to recover from heat cramps.

Get the victim out of the heat.

Loosen tight clothing.

Remove perspiration-soaked clothing.

Apply cool, wet cloths to the skin.

Fan the victim.

If victim is conscious, give cool water to drink.

Call for an ambulance if victim refuses water, vomits, or starts to lose consciousness.

carefully for further signals of heat-related illness.

Heat exhaustion is a more severe condition than heat cramps. It often affects athletes, fire fighters, construction workers, and factory workers, as well as those who wear heavy clothing in a hot, humid environment. Its signals include cool, moist, pale, or flushed skin, headache, nausea, dizziness, weakness, and exhaustion.

Heat stroke is the least common but most severe heat emergency. It most often occurs when people ignore the signals of heat exhaustion. Heat stroke develops when the body systems are overwhelmed by heat and begin to stop functioning. Heat stroke is a *serious* medical emergency. The signals of heat stroke include red, hot, dry skin; changes in consciousness; rapid, weak pulse; and rapid, shallow breathing.

When you recognize heat-related illness in its early stages, you can usually reverse it. Get the victim out of the heat. Loosen any tight clothing and apply cool, wet cloths, such as towels or sheets. If the victim is conscious, give cool water to drink.

Do not let the conscious victim drink too quickly. Give about one glass (4 ounces) of water every 15 minutes. Let the victim rest in a comfortable position, and watch carefully for changes in his or her condition. The victim should not resume normal activities the same day.

Refusing water, vomiting, and changes in consciousness mean that the victim's condition is getting worse. Call for an ambulance immediately if you have not already done so. If the victim vomits, stop giving fluids and position the victim on the side. Watch for signals of breathing problems. Keep the victim lying down and continue to cool the body any way you can. If you have ice packs or cold packs, place them on each of the victim's wrists and ankles, on the groin, in each armpit, and on the neck to cool the large blood vessels. *Do not* apply rubbing (isopropyl) alcohol.

Cold-Related Illness

Frostbite and hypothermia are two types of cold emergencies. Frostbite is the freezing of body parts exposed to the cold. Severity depends on the air temperature, length of exposure, and the wind. Frostbite can cause the loss of fingers, hands, arms, toes, feet, and legs.

The signals of frostbite include lack of feeling in the affected area and skin that appears waxy, is cold to the touch, or is discolored (flushed, white, yellow, or blue).

To care for any frostbite, handle the area gently. Never rub an affected area. Rubbing causes further damage to soft tissues. Instead, warm the area gently by soaking

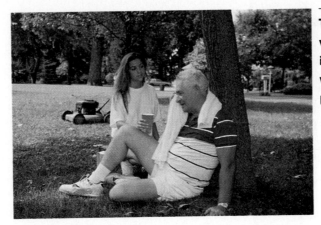

To cool the body of a victim of heat-related illness, cover with cool, wet towels and apply ice packs if necessary.

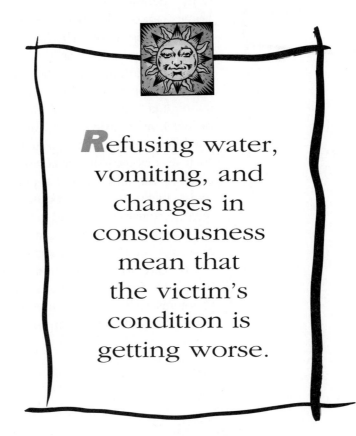

*R*efusing water, vomiting, and changes in consciousness mean that the victim's condition is getting worse.

the affected part in water no warmer than 105° F. If you don't have a thermometer, test the water temperature yourself. If the temperature is uncomfortable to your touch, the water is too warm. Keep the frostbitten part in the water until it looks red and feels warm. Loosely bandage the area with a dry, sterile dressing. If fingers or

> # The air temperature does not have to be below freezing for someone to get hypothermia.

toes are frostbitten, place cotton or gauze between them. Don't break any blisters. Get professional medical attention as soon as possible.

In hypothermia the entire body cools because its ability to keep warm fails. The victim will die if not given care. Signals of hypothermia include shivering, numbness, glassy stare, apathy, and loss of consciousness.

The air temperature does not have to be below freezing for people to develop hypothermia. Elderly people in poorly heated homes can develop hypothermia at higher temperatures. The homeless and the ill also are at risk. Substances that interfere with the body's normal response to cold, such as alcohol, may cause hypothermia to occur more easily. Any medical condition that impairs circulation, such as diabetes or cardiovascular disease, can also make a person more likely to get hypothermia. Anyone remaining in cold water or wet clothing for a long time may also easily develop hypothermia.

To care for hypothermia, start by caring for any life-threatening problems. Call the local emergency number. Make the victim comfort-able. Remove any wet clothing and dry the victim. Warm the body gradually by wrapping the victim in blankets or putting on dry clothing and moving him or her to a warm place. If they are available, apply heat pads or other heat sources to the body. Keep a barrier, such as a blanket, towel, or clothing, between the heat source and the victim to avoid burning him or her. If the victim is alert, give warm liquids to drink. Do not warm the victim too quickly, such as by immersing the victim in warm water. Rapid rewarming can cause dangerous heart problems. Handle the victim gently.

In cases of severe hypothermia the victim may be unconscious. Breathing might have slowed or stopped. The pulse may be slow and irregular. The body may feel stiff because the muscles become rigid. Call for an ambulance. Keep checking breathing and pulse. Give rescue breathing if necessary. Continue to warm the victim until EMS personnel arrive. Be prepared to start CPR.

In general, illnesses caused by overexposure to extreme temperatures can be prevented. To prevent heat or cold emergencies from hap-

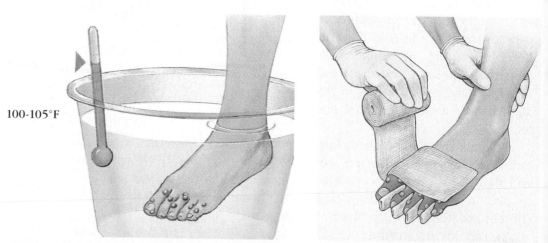

100-105°F

To care for frostbite, warm the frostbitten area by soaking the area in water (left). Do not allow the frostbitten area to touch the container. After rewarming, bandage the area with dry, sterile dressings. If fingers or toes are frostbitten, place gauze between them (right).

pening to you or anyone you know, follow these guidelines:

- Avoid being outdoors in the hottest or coldest part of the day.
- Change your activity level according to the temperature.
- Take frequent breaks.
- Dress appropriately for the environment.
- Drink large amounts of fluids.

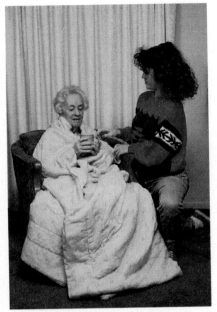

For a hypothermia victim, rewarm the body gradually by wrapping the victim in blankets or putting on dry clothing and moving him or her to a warm place.

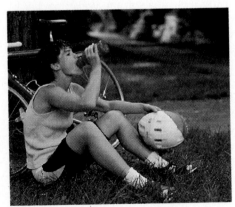

Taking frequent breaks when exercising in extreme temperatures allows your body to readjust to normal body temperature.

COLD-RELATED ILLNESS

Call for an ambulance.

Care for any life-threatening problems.

Move the victim to a warm place if you can.

Remove any wet clothing and dry the victim.

Warm the victim slowly by wrapping in blankets or putting on dry clothes.

Apply other sources of heat if they are available (chemical heat packs or hot water bottles).

FYI

The High-Tech War Against Cold

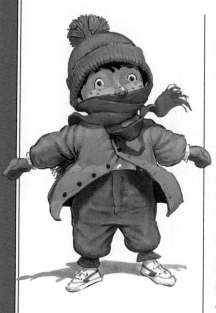

REFERENCES
1. Recreation Equipment Incorporated. *Layering for Comfort: FYI, An Informational Brochure from REI.* Seattle, WA, 1991.
2. Recreation Equipment Incorporated. *Understanding Outdoor Fabrics: FYI, An Informational Brochure from REI.* Seattle, WA, 1991.

In the past, we depended entirely on nature for clothing. Animal skins, furs, and feathers protected us from freezing temperatures. As long as seasonal changes and cold climates exist, preventing cold-related illnesses, such as hypothermia, remains important when we work or play outside. Although natural fibers, such as wool and down, are still very useful, a whole family of synthetic fibers is now used to make clothing. Being outdoors has become a lot more comfortable.

The best way to use outdoor fabrics is to layer them. This creates warmth by trapping warm air between layers to insulate the body. Layering is an old concept: wear several layers of clothing when it's cold; take clothes off when warm and put them back on if you get cold. This enables you to regulate your body temperature and deal with changes in the environment.

Start off with an underwear layer. Commonly called long underwear, it includes thin, snug-fitting pants and a long-sleeved shirt. Underwear should supply you with basic insulation and pull moisture away from your skin—damp, sweaty skin can chill you when you slow down or stop. Natural fibers, such as cotton, wool, and silk, can be quite warm and are okay for light activity. For heavier exercise, however, synthetic fabrics absorb less moisture and actually carry water droplets away from your skin. Polypropylene and Capilene are two popular synthetic fabrics for underwear.

Next, add one or more insulating layers such as a wool sweater or a down jacket, depending on the temperature. Don't forget your legs. Wool pants are a better choice than jeans or corduroys. Synthetic materials used in jackets and pants include Thinsulate, Qualofil, and pile (a plush, nonpiling polyester fiber). Although down is an excellent, lightweight insulator, it becomes useless when wet, so a quick-drying fabric-like pile may keep you warmer in a damp climate.

Finish with a windproof, and preferably waterproof, shell layer. Synthetic, high-tech fabrics make a strong showing here. Windproof fabrics wear names like Supplex, Silmond, Captiva, or ripstop nylon. Coatings, such as Hypalon, applied to jackets and pants are completely water-repellent. However, the newest waterproof fabrics are "breathable." They repel wind and rain but allow your perspiration to pass through the fabric so that you stay dry and warmer. Gore-Tex, Thintech, Ultrex, and Super Microft are some of the names given to these fabrics. Check your shell for wind seals at the waist, neck, wrists, and ankles and make sure it is big enough to fit several layers of clothing underneath.

A hat is vital to staying truly warm. Gloves, insulating socks, neck "gaiters," and headbands all protect you from the cold. Visit your local outdoor store for more information about the best clothing for your specific work or recreation.

Layering clothing allows the wearer to regulate body temperature and deal with changes in weather. Clothing layers can be used in combination or separately, depending on the climate and activity.

Inner Layer

Recreational Equipment Inc.

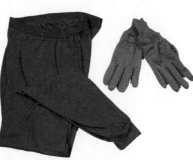

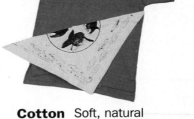

Capilene Lightweight, synthetic fabric that doesn't absorb moisture. Designed to pull moisture away from skin where it can evaporate.

Cotton Soft, natural fibers that absorb moisture and allow air to circulate.

Insulating Layer

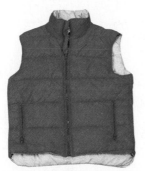

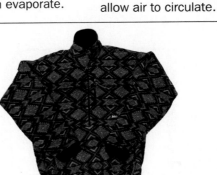

Qualofil Exceptionally warm, wet or dry.

Pile Soft, polyester fabric that is warmer per pound than wool. Insulates when wet and is quick drying.

Shell Layer

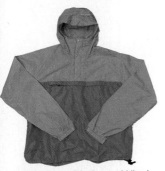

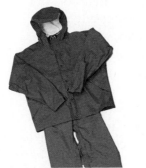

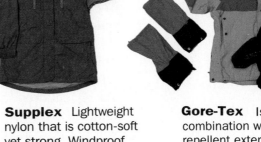

Ripstop Nylon Windproof, resistant to moisture, and has some breathability. Protects against fog, light rain, snow.

Hypalon Versatile, synthetic rubber applied to lightweight nylon is completely water-repellent. Unaffected by saltwater and highly resistant to abrasion.

Supplex Lightweight nylon that is cotton-soft yet strong. Windproof, breathable, some water repellancy, quick drying.

Gore-Tex Is used in combination with water repellent exterior fabric. Allows perspiration to escape while preventing water and wind from seeping in.

THE YOUNG AND THE ELDERLY

Caring for an ill or injured child is not always easy, especially if it is a child you do not know. Children are not simply small adults. They have unique needs and require special care. Some children do not readily accept strangers. This can make it difficult to accurately check a child's condition. Young children can be especially difficult to check, since they often will not be able to tell you what is wrong.

It is often difficult to imagine how a young child with a serious

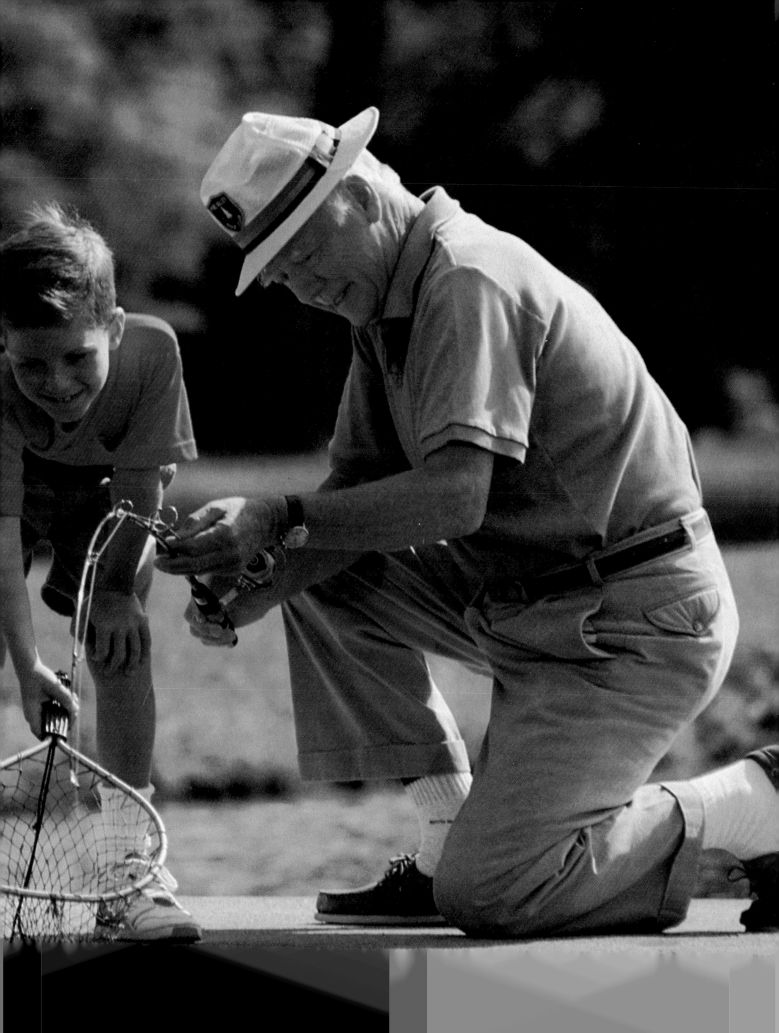

illness or injury feels. One of a child's main emotions is fear. The fears that a child experiences are real. A child is afraid of the unknown. He or she is afraid of being ill or hurt, of being touched by strangers, and of being separated from his or her parents. How you interact with a child is very important. You need to try to reduce anxiety and panic in the child.

Children up to 1 year of age are commonly referred to as infants. Young infants, those less than 6 months old, are relatively easy to approach. Your presence will not generally bother children of this age group. Older infants, however,

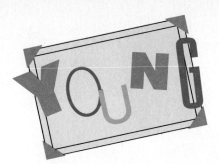

Kids have unique needs that require special care.

will often exhibit "stranger anxiety." They are uncomfortable around strangers and may cry and cling to a parent or guardian.

Children 1 and 2 years of age are called toddlers. These children are frequently uncooperative. A toddler will be concerned that he

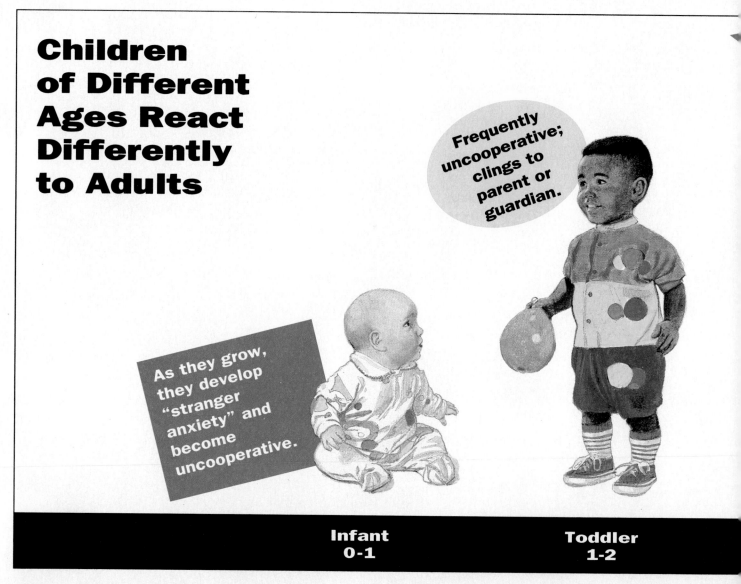

Children of Different Ages React Differently to Adults

Frequently uncooperative; clings to parent or guardian.

As they grow, they develop "stranger anxiety" and become uncooperative.

Infant
0-1

Toddler
1-2

or she will be separated from the parent or guardian. Reassurance that this will not happen will often comfort a concerned child of this age. It is often best to check a toddler in the parent's or guardian's lap.

Children aged 3, 4, and 5 are generally referred to as preschoolers. Children in this age group are usually easy to check if approached properly. Use their natural curiosity. Allow them to inspect items such as bandages.

School-aged children are those between 6 and 12 years of age. They are usually cooperative and can be a good source of informa-

tion about what happened. You should be able to talk with them readily. Children in this age group are becoming conscious of their bodies. Respect the child's modesty.

Adolescents are between 13 and 18 years of age. They are typically more like an adult than a child. Direct your questions to them instead of to parents or guardians. However, allow input from a parent or

guardian. Occasionally, in the presence of a parent or guardian, it may not be possible to get an accurate idea of what happened or what is wrong. Also adolescents are modest and often respond better to a caregiver of the same gender.

Kids Have Special Problems

Injury remains the number one cause of death for children in the

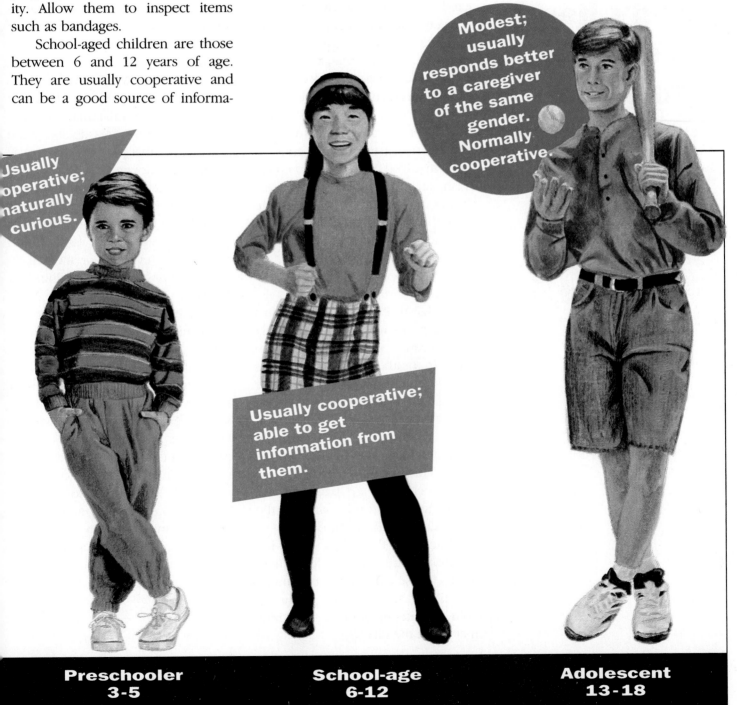

Usually cooperative; naturally curious.

Usually cooperative; able to get information from them.

Modest; usually responds better to a caregiver of the same gender. Normally cooperative.

Preschooler 3-5

School-age 6-12

Adolescent 13-18

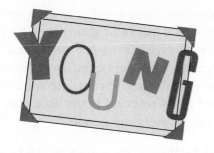

Because a child's head is usually large in proportion to the body, the head is often injured.

United States. Many of these deaths are the result of motor vehicle crashes. The greatest dangers to a child involved in a vehicle incident that results in serious injury are a blocked airway and bleeding. Because a child's head is usually large in proportion to the rest of the body, the head is often injured.

To avoid some of the needless deaths of children associated with motor vehicles, laws have been enacted requiring that children ride in safety seats or wear safety belts. As a result, more lives will be saved.

You may have to check and care for an injured child while he or she is in a car seat. A car seat does not normally pose any problem when you are trying to check a child. A child involved in a motor vehicle crash and found in a car seat should be left in the seat if the device has not been damaged. If the child is to be transported to a medical facility for evaluation, he or she can be easily secured in the car seat.

A high fever in a child indicates some type of infection. In a young child, even a minor infection can result in a rather high fever. This is often defined as a temperature above 103° F. Prolonged or excessively high fever can result in seizures. Your initial care for a child with high fever is to gently cool the child. This includes removing excessive clothing or blankets and sponging lukewarm water on the child. Call the doctor at once.

Infections that affect breathing are more common in children than adults. These can range from minor infections, such as the common cold, to life-threatening infections that block the airway.

One such illness is croup. Croup is an infection that causes swelling of the throat below the vocal cords. Besides the basic signals of breathing problems and a cough that sounds like the bark of a seal, croup is often preceded by 1 or 2 days of illness, sometimes with a fever. Croup occurs more often in the winter months, and the signals are often evident in the evening. It generally is not life-threatening. The child will often improve when exposed to cool air, such as the air outdoors, or cool steam from a vaporizer.

Another childhood problem is epiglottitis. This is an infection that causes a severe inflammation of the epiglottis, a flap of tissue above the vocal cords that protects the airway during swallowing. When it becomes infected, the epiglottis can swell to a point where the airway is completely blocked. The child with epiglottitis will appear quite ill and have a high fever. He or she will often be sitting up and straining to breathe. The child will be very frightened. Saliva may be drooling from his or her mouth because swelling of the epiglottis prevents the child from swallowing.

You will not need to distinguish between croup and epiglottitis, since the care you provide will be the same for either situation. To care for a child who is having trouble breathing, allow him or her to remain in the most comfortable position for breathing. Do not attempt to place any object in the child's mouth. Call the child's doctor at once. If this is not possible, call your local emergency number for

CHECKING A CHILD

Checking an ill or injured child can be a challenge, especially if you do not know him or her. The following are a few basic guidelines that will help you.

Observe the Child Before Touching Him or Her
You can find out much information before you actually touch the child. Look for signals that indicate changes in consciousness, any breathing difficulty, and any apparent injuries or conditions. All may change as soon as you touch the child because he or she may become anxious or upset.

Remain Calm
Caring for ill or injured children can be very stressful. Staying calm will show confidence and help keep the child and parent or guardian calm.

Communicate Clearly with the Parent or Guardian and the Child
If the family is excited or agitated, the child is likely to be so too. When you can calm the family, the child will often calm down as well. Explain what you wish to do. Get at eye level with the child. Talk slowly and use simple words when speaking with the child. Ask questions that can be easily answered.

Do Not Separate the Child from Loved Ones Unless Necessary
This is especially true for younger children (under age 7 or 8). Often a parent or guardian will be holding a crying child. In this case, you can check the child while the parent or guardian continues to hold him or her.

Gain Trust Through Your Actions
Explain what you are going to do before you do it. Be sure to use terms and language the child will understand. Check a conscious child from the feet to the head rather than head to toe. The child is more likely to accept you first touching the feet and progressing to the head. You should still look and feel for the same things.

an ambulance. If the child's airway becomes completely blocked as a result of epiglottitis, there is nothing you can do to help; this child needs professional help. Call for an ambulance immediately.

Older Adults

The elderly are generally considered those over 65 years of age. They are quickly becoming the fastest growing population group in the United States. A major reason is

MEMO

"Joe, I'm really beginning to worry about your dad. At first it was just little things—like forgetting where he put his glasses and what day it was, and how to work the VCR, but now it's worse. Last week he went out and Mrs. Chung found him wandering the street and brought him home. He couldn't remember where he lived or who he was! Yesterday he just walked out while we were talking. Later, he didn't remember anything about it. It's not safe for him to be out by himself anymore. Maybe there's something that will make him better. I just don't know what I'm going to do!"

Joe's dad needs several medical examinations to try to determine the reasons for his memory decline. Perhaps he has a condition that can be reversed or helped. But the chances are high that he has a condition known as Alzheimer's disease. At one time considered a rare disorder, today Alzheimer's disease (AD) is the most common cause of dementia. Dementia is the loss of intellectual functions such as thinking, remembering, and reasoning, which is severe enough to interfere with a person's daily activities.

AD affects an estimated 4 million American adults and results in 100,000 deaths annually. Most victims are over 65; however, AD can strike people in their 40s and 50s. Men and women are affected almost equally.[1] At this time, scientists are still looking for the cause of AD. A confirmed diagnosis of the disease can only be made by examining the victim's brain tissue after death. And while there are no treatments to stop or reverse the mental decline from AD, several drugs are available now to help manage some of the symptoms.

Signals of AD develop gradually. They include confusion, progressive memory loss, and changes in personality, behavior, and the ability to think and communicate. Eventually, victims of AD become totally unable to care for themselves.[2]

There are a number of disorders that have symptoms similar to those of AD. Some of them can be treated. Therefore, it is very important that anyone who is experiencing memory loss or confusion has a thorough medical examination.

an increase in life expectancy because of improvements in health care. Since 1900, there has been a 53 percent increase in life expectancy. For example, in 1900, the average life expectancy was 49 years. Today the average life expectancy is over 75 years.

Many changes occur with age. Overall, there is a general decline in body function, with some changes beginning as early as age 30. Both the heart and lungs suffer the effects of aging. The amount of blood pumped by the heart with each beat decreases and the heart rate slows. The blood vessels harden, causing increased work for the heart. The

Most people with illnesses such as AD are cared for by their families for much of their illness. Providing care at home requires careful planning. The home has to be made safe, and routines set up for daily activities such as mealtimes, personal care, and leisure.

Services That Help

It is important for anyone caring for a person with Alzheimer's, or a related problem, to realize that they are not alone. There are people and organizations that can help both you and the person with AD. For health care services, a physician, perhaps your family doctor or a specialist, can give you medical advice, including help with difficult behavior and personality changes.

If you are caring for an AD victim living at home, you may need help with some basic services such as nutrition and transportation. A visiting nurse or nutritionist can help you, and a volunteer program like Meals on Wheels may be helpful. Volunteer or paid transportation services may also be available to take AD victims to and from health facilities, day care, and other programs.

Visiting nurses, home health aides, and homemakers can come to your home and provide help with health care, bathing and dressing, shopping, and cooking. Many adult day care centers provide recreational activities designed for people with AD. Some hospitals, nursing homes, and other facilities may take in AD victims for short stays. For AD victims who can no longer live at home, group homes or foster homes may be available. Nursing homes offer more skilled nursing and some specialize in the care of victims of AD or similar diseases. A few hospice programs accept AD victims who are nearing the end of their life. Explore to find out which, if any, services are covered by Medicare, Medicaid, Social Security disability, or veterans' benefits in your state. A lawyer or a social worker may be able to help you.

To locate services that can help you, the AD victim, and other family members, check the yellow pages under Social Service Organizations and state and local government listings in the phone directory. Places you can call for information include your local health department, office on aging, and department of social services or senior citizen's services. Churches, synagogues, and other religious institutions may also have information and programs; so may senior centers and nursing home staffs, hospital geriatric departments, doctors, nurses, social workers, and counselors. Your location may have a chapter of the Alzheimer's Association nearby. To locate a chapter near you, call the Association's 24-hour, toll-free number: 1-800-272-3900. This organization has chapters and support groups across the country where you can get information and guidance.

REFERENCES
1. Alzheimer's Disease and Related Disorders Association, Inc. *Alzheimer's Disease Fact Sheet*, 1990.
2. Alzheimer's Disease and Related Disorders Association, Inc. *If You Think Someone You Know Has Alzheimer's Disease*, 1990.
3. Alzheimer's Disease and Related Disorders Association, Inc. *Alzheimer's Disease: Services You May Need*, 1990.

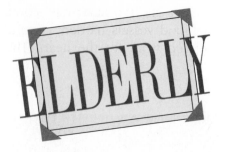

Older adults are more prone to injury and illness as body functions generally decline.

number of working brain cells also decreases with age. Hearing and vision usually decline, often causing some degree of sight and hearing loss. Reflexes become slower, and arthritis may affect joints, causing movement to become painful.

As a result of slower reflexes, failing eyesight and hearing, arthritis, and problems related to the blood vessels, such as numbness, the elderly are at increased risk of injury from falls. Falls frequently result in fractures because the bones become weaker and more brittle with age.

An elderly person is also at greater risk of serious head injuries. This is mainly because as we age, the size of the brain decreases. This results in more space between the surface of the brain and the inside of the skull. This space allows more movement of the brain within the skull, which can increase the likelihood of serious head injury. Occasionally, an elderly person may not develop the signals of a head injury until days after a fall. Therefore, you should always suspect a head injury as a possible cause of unusual behavior in an elderly person, especially if the victim has had a fall or blow to the head.

The elderly are also prone to problems with the nervous system, especially stroke. In addition, the elderly are at increased risk of altered thinking patterns and confusion. Some change is a result of aging. However, certain diseases occurring in some elderly persons also cause problems with the way the mind works. The most common of these is Alzheimer's disease, a disease that affects the brain. It results in impaired memory, thinking, and behavior. Alzheimer's affects an estimated 2.5 million adults.

If you are providing care for an elderly person who is confused, try to find out whether the confusion is the result of injury or a condition the victim already has. Get at the victim's eye level so he or she can see and hear you more clearly. Sometimes confusion is actually the result of decreased vision or hearing.

Your care for the elderly victim requires you to keep in mind the special problems and concerns of the elderly and to communicate appropriately. Often, an elderly victim's problem will seem unimportant to him or her. He or she may not recognize the signals of a serious condition. The victim may also downplay signals out of fear of losing his or her independence or of being placed in a nursing home. Do not talk down to an elderly person, as you would a child. In some circumstances, you should gather the victim's medications and see that they are with the victim if he or she is being taken to a medical facility.

INDEX